THE DASH DIET COOKBOOK

JOHN CHATHAM

ROCKRIDGE UNIVERSITY PRESS

CONTENTS

INTRODUCTION

D o you really want to entrust your health to a fad? Do you know if any of the diet plans in books or on the Internet really work? Do you trust any of the diets out there?

It's difficult enough admitting that you need and want help controlling your weight and your health. What makes it even more challenging is that there is so much conflicting information about how to go about losing weight and gaining back one's good health. Picked by *US News & World Report* as its number-one choice in Best Diets Overall, Best Diets for Healthy Eating, and Best Diabetes Diets, the DASH diet rises above the noise of the gimmicky weight-loss plans year after year. The DASH diet is nutritionally sound, based on extensive scientific research, and has received widespread support and approval from the health and medical communities. On the DASH diet, you won't starve or feel deprived, and best of all, you'll be lowering your blood pressure and cholesterol levels; reducing your risk of heart disease, diabetes, and stroke; and losing weight, all while enjoying rosemary chicken, seafood fettuccine, and more.

This medically developed plan works because it was designed primarily to improve one's health. Instead of being stuck in the diet doldrums, you will feel satisfied and full of energy, because the DASH diet isn't about eating less food—it's about eating the right foods for optimal health.

The DASH Diet Cookbook includes streamlined program details so you can get started on the diet right away, and best of all, it includes more than a hundred DASH diet recipes designed with your taste buds *and* your health in mind.

SECTION ONE
The DASH Diet Basics

1

WHAT YOU NEED TO KNOW ABOUT THE DASH DIET

The History of the DASH Diet

In response to the growing problem of high blood pressure in the United States, the National Institutes of Health (NIH) provided funding in 1992 for research into a dietary solution to hypertension. The goal was to create Dietary Approaches to Stop Hypertension (DASH).

The National Heart, Lung, and Blood Institute (NHLBI) conducted this research with the help of five of the most respected medical research institutions in the country. Together, these five facilities conducted the most extensive and exhaustive research to date on nutritional solutions for the growing problem of hypertension.

Teams of doctors, nutritionists, nurses, and statisticians worked cooperatively between their respective institutions on randomized control trials. Each facility chose and studied its own groups of participants to ensure the most accurate research results. More than eight thousand people went through the screening process, and the researchers specifically sought to fill at least two-thirds of the spots with people at high risk of hypertension.

Two DASH trials were conducted in all. By the end of the second study, the results showed that a diet consisting of high fiber, low-fat dairy, plenty of fresh fruits and vegetables, lean protein, plus lower sodium and sugar intake produced blood pressure reduction in people who were considered prehypertensive. The hypertensive participants had an even higher reduction. These results were apparent after just thirty days on the DASH diet.

These studies, along with additional research, showed that the DASH diet not only reduced blood pressure but cholesterol and body fat, particularly around the abdomen. These findings are the reason that the DASH diet is recommended by medical organizations such as the American Medical Association, the American Heart Association, and many others.

The 2012 Dietary Guidelines for Americans recommend the DASH eating plan for everyone, including children and the elderly. The DASH diet even formed the basis for the MyPlate dietary guidelines (the new food pyramid) generated by the United States Department of Agriculture (USDA).

An Overview of the DASH Diet Plan

- **Reduces sodium to lower hypertension** or the risk of hypertension. Choose the standard DASH diet that allows up to 2,300 milligrams (mg) of sodium per day or a low-sodium version that allows up to 1,500 mg of sodium per day. The typical American diet includes as much as 3,500 mg of sodium per day!
- **Increases fiber to reduce blood pressure,** steady blood sugar levels, and aid in weight loss. The DASH diet provides more fresh fruits and vegetables than most people are used to eating, as well as a healthful selection of whole grains.

- **Reduces saturated fat and trans fat** in order to increase heart health, lower LDL (bad) cholesterol, raise HDL (good) cholesterol, aid in weight loss, and decrease risks and symptoms of heart disease, diabetes, and metabolic syndrome. Trans fats (from processed and fried foods) are omitted, and foods low in saturated fats, such as low-fat dairy, lean meats, and seafood, are encouraged.
- **Increases healthful fats** by eating nuts, seeds, fish, avocado, and other Omega-3–rich foods.
- **Helps reduce blood pressure** by limiting alcohol and caffeine.
- **Ensures proper levels of the minerals** shown to reduce high blood pressure, such as potassium and magnesium. Eating a wide variety of foods containing minerals, such as bananas, legumes (beans), and leafy greens, boosts mineral intake.
- **Reduces the risk of type 2 diabetes** and metabolic syndrome while lowering abdominal fat (a leading indicator of both). Sugary foods are limited to no more than five per week.

The DASH Diet's Effect on Your Health

Unlike most diet plans, the DASH diet wasn't created as a means of losing weight; it was designed to reduce high blood pressure, which in turn helps prevent heart disease and stroke.

The DASH Diet and High Blood Pressure

Following the DASH diet plan—particularly the low-sodium version of the diet—has been shown to have a direct impact on high blood pressure. This combination of specific nutrients with a low sodium intake has produced significant positive results in every major study conducted.

If you're at a high risk of developing high blood pressure due to your ethnicity (African Americans are in this high-risk group), lifestyle choices (such as smoking and high sodium intake), or weight (obesity is a leading indicator of hypertension risk), the DASH diet is the recommended diet for reducing your risk.

The DASH Diet and Type 2 Diabetes

It has been shown that the symptoms and severity of type 2 diabetes can be greatly lessened with a DASH-style diet, and that the condition can sometimes even be reversed with these dietary changes.

All of the foods included in the DASH diet are recommended to help improve the health of those with type 2 diabetes, but some are particularly effective. Nuts can improve glucose control in diabetics. Similarly, the high fiber content of the diet works to slow the absorption of sugar, which helps to prevent serious swings in blood sugar levels. The high level of antioxidants in all the DASH-recommended fresh fruits and vegetables can also help to prevent or reduce type 2 diabetes complications.

One of the most important ways that the DASH diet can help those with or at risk for type 2 diabetes is in weight loss. Excess body fat—particularly abdominal fat—is one of the biggest contributors to insulin insensitivity. It also further increases the risk of heart disease for diabetics.

The DASH Diet and Metabolic Syndrome

Metabolic syndrome serves as an umbrella term for a group of obesity- and insulin-related symptoms. The syndrome is commonly referred to as "prediabetes" because it often leads to type 2 diabetes if it isn't corrected.

The typical diagnostic markers of metabolic syndrome include a large waist size, high fasting glucose (blood sugar) levels, high triglycerides, and elevated HDL cholesterol. DASH's lowered intake of bad fats and increased intake of good fats and fiber helps to lower HDL cholesterol and triglyceride levels. The nutrients you'll consume on the DASH diet, coupled with significant fat loss around the abdomen, can reverse, prevent, or significantly reduce metabolic syndrome.

The DASH Diet and Heart Disease

People with high blood pressure, type 2 diabetes, and metabolic syndrome have a high risk of developing heart disease. Since the DASH diet addresses these conditions, it in turn addresses your risk for heart disease.

Heart disease is the leading cause of death in America, and health professionals have long known that a diet low in unhealthful fats and high in healthful fats and fiber will positively impact heart health. As a result, the DASH diet has gained the support of the American Heart Association because of its heart-healthful diet.

In addition to the benefits for your heart, the DASH diet has also been credited with lowering the risk of kidney stones and improving digestive and colon health; your heart won't be the only beneficiary of a DASH eating plan!

Fat Intake and Weight Loss

The DASH diet is far lower in fat than the typical American diet. It reduces or eliminates unhealthful fats, which includes fried foods, fast food, and highly processed foods. However, healthful fats such as unsaturated fats and omega-3 fats, which are good for your body, are allowed.

Fiber Intake and Weight Loss

The DASH diet is rich in soluble and insoluble fiber, which help you to feel full, aid in efficient digestion, and slow the absorption of fat and sugar into your bloodstream. This slowed absorption rate aids in weight loss by helping your body regulate and respond to insulin more efficiently.

Vitamin C and Weight Loss

Because the DASH diet is so high in fresh fruits and vegetables, you will consume a wide range of essential vitamins, minerals, and antioxidants. One of the most important of these nutrients is vitamin C.

In recent years, a great deal of research has come out about the value of vitamin C in fat loss. Vitamin C reduces the effects of stress on the body, which in turn reduces the amount of cortisol (the stress hormone) that is released into the bloodstream. Cortisol's main function is to aid in the storage of fat around the abdomen as a biological insurance policy against famine. When you reduce the amount of stress in your life, you reduce the amount of cortisol that is released into your system. This means that less of what you eat will end up stored in your abdomen.

Calorie Intake and Weight Loss

For years, the mainstream approach to weight loss was "if you take in fewer calories than you burn, you'll lose weight." Current research shows that reducing calories *can* result in weight loss, but this alone will not necessarily result in fat loss. This can result in the loss of lean muscle tissue and water instead of stored fat.

The DASH diet prescribes a caloric intake that varies from participant to participant. This intake takes your current weight, weight-loss goals, activity level, and body type into consideration—a process that is covered in the next chapter.

An All-Around Healthful Plan for Weight Loss Success

The DASH diet incorporates multiple healthful eating strategies, providing a nutritionally sound method for weight loss. With this realistic, delicious, and healthful eating plan, DASH participants have found that they are more likely to reach their weight-loss goals and make a permanent lifestyle change for the better.

Additional Benefits

- You can easily find DASH-friendly food options when eating at restaurants or a friend's house.
- Once you've reached your ideal weight, the realistic methods of DASH make it easier to maintain.
- You have the option to choose a sodium level that is appropriate for you.
- The DASH diet outlines how you can increase or decrease your caloric intake as your activity level and body mass change.
- It is simple to adapt popular recipes to fit the DASH diet.

2

PLANNING YOUR DASH DIET

Good preparation is essential to making any new endeavor successful. You need to know that you have the right tools and supplies—and that your goals are realistic—before you get started.

The DASH diet isn't difficult or complicated, but it will likely cause a significant change to your lifestyle. Being successful on the DASH diet requires commitment, determination, and a bit of planning to avoid the pitfalls that might cause discouragement or frustration.

What Is Your Body Mass Index?

The first thing that you need to do is establish your health and fitness goals. Most people rely on the bathroom scale to tell them how much weight they need to lose, but that's really not the most accurate measurement.

Start by determining your *body mass index* (BMI). This index approximates the percentage of your body weight that is fat. You can get your body fat calculated by professionals or purchase a body fat measurement kit; alternately, you can get a fairly accurate measurement of your BMI with a measuring tape and an online calculator.

Next, measure your weight. To do this, you'll need to weigh yourself first thing in the morning, after urinating and before eating or drinking. Wear only your underwear or nothing at all. Record your weight in the appropriate blank on the *BMI Assessment Form* at the end of this chapter.

Next, you'll need to gather some measurements to use in calculating your BMI. For men, measure the circumference of your neck and abdomen. Be sure the measuring tape keeps in contact with your skin without pulling it too tightly. To measure your abdomen, wrap the measuring tape around your body at a point just below your belly button. For women, measure the circumference of your neck, waist, and hips. Measure your waist at the slimmest point of your torso, and measure your hips just below the hipbones; the measuring tape should cross the top portion of your buttocks. As you take these measurements, write them down on the *BMI Assessment Form* at the end of this chapter.

Once you have your measurements, you can calculate your BMI using one of the many free calculators that are available online. One calculator you can use is: http://www.linear-software.com/online.html.

Enter the value on the "Body Fat %" line of the *BMI Assessment Form*.

With an understanding of your body fat percentage, you can begin understanding your current state of health and have a point of comparison after you have started following the DASH diet. While you can weigh yourself along the way and celebrate pounds lost, recalculating your BMI is often a more efficient way to track your progress.

If you follow the DASH diet as well as exercise regularly, you'll likely be gaining lean muscle mass as you lose fat. In this situation, a scale can't tell the difference between muscle weight and fat weight; lean muscle weighs more than fat but is more compact than fat tissue. As a result, the scale may say you've gained weight, but you are likely to see an improvement in your BMI. To see an example of this improvement in action, return to the BMI calculator you used for your initial calculation and reduce your measurements by several inches (just one or two inches at the neck, and a few to several inches at the waist, abdomen, or hips). This will show the change in your BMI, given those hypothetical measurements.

What Is Your Basal Metabolic Rate?

Once you have an understanding of your BMI, it is important to calculate the number of calories that your body requires to maintain your current weight. This calculation will help you understand the number of calories you should consume in order to lose weight at a safe and comfortable pace.

To perform this calculation, you will first calculate your *basal metabolic rate* or BMR. The BMR formula takes your height, weight, age, and gender into account in its calculation. This method is likely to be more accurate than calculating your calorie needs based solely on body weight. Since leaner bodies burn more calories than less lean ones, this method will be accurate unless you are very muscular or very obese. If you're very fit and muscular, you may need to add more calories, and if you're very overweight, you may need to deduct them. Trial and error will help you make these types of adjustments as you progress in your diet.

The following formula will calculate your BMR:

- **For Women**: BMR = 655 + (4.35 x weight in pounds) + (4.7 x height in inches) − (4.7 x age in years)
- **For Men**: BMR = 66 + (6.23 x weight in pounds) + (12.7 x height in inches) − (6.8 x age in years)

Calculate your BMR and record it in on the *BMI Assessment Form* at the end of this chapter.

What Are Your Daily Calorie Requirements?

In order to determine your *daily calorie requirements* (DCR) you'll need to factor in your activity level. To do this, we use what is known as the *Harris Benedict Equation.*

To determine your total daily calorie needs, multiply your BMR by the appropriate activity factor, as follows:

- If you are sedentary (little or no exercise):
  Calorie Calculation = BMR x 1.2

- If you are lightly active (exercise 1–3 days/week):
  Calorie Calculation = BMR x 1.375

- If you are moderately active (exercise 3–5 days/week):
  Calorie Calculation = BMR x 1.55

- If you are very active (6–7 days/week):
  Calorie Calculation = BMR x 1.725

- If you are extra active (exercise and physical job or double training):
  Calorie Calculation = BMR x 1.9

Calculate your BMR and record it on the *BMI Assessment Form* at the end of this chapter.

Once you know the number of calories needed to maintain your weight, you can easily calculate the number of calories you need to eat in order to gain or lose weight:

One pound equals 3,500 calories, so to lose one pound a week you would deduct 500 calories from your total daily caloric requirements (not your BMR). To lose two pounds a week, you would need to deduct 1,000 calories per day.

For people whose daily caloric requirement is low, trying to lose weight solely by cutting calories may be impractical and unsustainable. It's healthful to combine increased activity and decreased calorie intake, but this is especially true for those who already have a low calorie requirement.

You can start out using the caloric requirements for your present activity level, minus 500–1,000 calories per day. In two weeks, if you're staying on schedule with a fitness program, recalculate your daily calorie needs using the appropriate new activity level. This will ensure that you're getting enough nutrition yet still staying on track for your weight loss.

BMI Assessment Form

Date ....

Weight ....

Neck ....

Waist .... (Women)

Hips .... (Women)

Abdomen .... (Men)

Body Fat % ....

BMR: .... calories

DCR: ....

Note: You might want to copy several blank assessment forms to help track your progress until you reach your goals.

(3)

TRANSITIONING TO THE DASH DIET

The decision to take on a new diet is difficult, one that will require discipline and hard work. Once you commit to incorporating the DASH diet into your lifestyle, it is essential to properly prepare for your journey toward health.

Here are some important steps and tips that you should integrate into your lifestyle at least one week before you officially start the DASH diet.

Clean House

One of the best things you can do to achieve success is to eliminate all of the off-limits foods from the house. You know your own weaknesses better than anyone, so even if something is allowed on the DASH diet food list, get rid of it if you know it is an item you will have a hard time consuming in moderation.

Plan Your Menu Ahead of Time

The key to achieving success with the DASH diet is to plan your meals in advance. Preparation of meal plans helps with shopping, prepares you for a new way of eating, and eliminates unhealthful snacking once you begin the diet.

Prepare Your Taste Buds

The week before you start your diet, begin to cut back on portion sizes, take the saltshaker off the table, opt for fruit when it comes to dessert, and skip the junk food. By the time you start your diet, your body will already be in the process of adjusting to this new way of eating (and intense cravings will have diminished).

Start an Exercise Plan a Week Early or a Week Late

Starting a new diet and a new workout program at the same time can be overwhelming. If you thrive on that kind of radical change, then go ahead and do it. If not, start your exercise plan the week before or after you begin the DASH diet.

The Top 10 Tips to Success

1. Trade in Your Saltshaker

Plan ahead and eliminate salt whenever you can, so you can enjoy it in other foods where it cannot be eliminated. This is especially important if you have high blood pressure and need to follow the lowest sodium version of the diet. Whenever possible, use salt substitutes or another herb blend in place of salt.

2. Make the Right Choices the Easiest Ones

Make sure that fresh fruits and other healthful snacks, such as dark chocolate and sorbet, are more visible than tempting treats. To ward off temptation, keep healthful snacks and a water bottle accessible, and avoid the fast-food lunch trap by bringing your own meals to work.

3. Exercise First Thing in the Morning

Something always gets in the way of exercise, especially when a new workout routine is being initiated. Until you're hooked on fitness, and not inclined to use any excuse that comes your way to avoid exercise, it is best to work out as soon as you wake up. It's always possible to change your workout schedule, but wait until working out has become a habit. (Usually, this takes about thirty days.)

4. Drink a Ton of Water

Most experts recommend drinking at least sixty-four ounces of water per day. If you're not already doing this, you need to start. Your new diet is full of foods that aid digestion, but you need a lot of water to get things moving. Adequate water will also help you to lose excess stored water, feel fuller longer, and have more energy.

5. Skip Restaurants for the First Two Weeks

While you shouldn't deprive yourself of things you enjoy, like going out to eat, it's better to wait until you're used to making healthier choices, and seeing results that motivate you to stick with the diet.

6. Buddy-Up, or Get Your Friends to Support You

If possible, enlist a family member or friend to go on the diet with you. Getting someone to join you for workouts can also be a big help.

7. Enjoy Eating

The recipes in this book are tools to guide you and help you follow the DASH diet. If you're not enjoying your food, you won't be on the diet for very long.

8. Keep a Journal

Keep a small notebook handy and jot down your progress. Write down what you eat and how you feel after, or your thoughts on achieving a good workout or winning a battle against temptation. These notes can really help keep you motivated, especially when you hit a rough patch.

9. Avoid or Plan for Food Triggers

Most people have certain triggers that result in overeating or making poor food choices. Identify your triggers and figure out ways to avoid them altogether, or at least outwit them.

10. Circumvent Stress Eating

Stress-induced eating is a common problem. It's easy to justify eating during stressful moments, which is why it is important to develop an emergency plan of action before you face the situation. Identify stress-alleviating alternatives in advance, such as going on a short walk or calling a good friend, and follow through with the plan when you recognize your stress levels rising.

(4)

YOUR DASH DIET EATING PLAN

The DASH diet is a roadmap toward a healthier lifestyle. The flexibility of the diet is designed to enable you to make necessary changes as easily as possible. As your health and fitness improves, modify the program to fit your personal needs. It's easy to see why millions of people (even those who don't yet have any health problems) have chosen the DASH diet to improve their health and lose excess weight and fat.

The DASH Diet Food List

Meats and Seafood

Allowed:

- All fish, especially salmon, haddock, mackerel, sardines, and other oily fish
- All shellfish
- Beef: lean steaks and roasts, leanest possible ground meat
- Chicken, skinless
- Eggs
- Game birds
- Game meats

- Lamb: lean stew meat, steaks, and roasts
- Pork: lean steaks and roasts
- Turkey: skinless and ground breast meat
- Venison

Not Allowed:

- Bacon, except for low-salt turkey bacon
- Jerky
- Packaged cold cuts and deli meats
- Sausage

Dairy

Allowed:

- Almond milk
- Blue cheese
- Cheddar cheese (reduced fat)
- Cow's milk (1 percent or nonfat)
- Cream cheese (reduced fat)
- Feta cheese
- Greek yogurt
- Cottage cheese (low or nonfat)
- Margarine or butter substitute
- Mozzarella cheese
- Parmesan cheese (high sodium, so limit quantities)
- Provolone cheese (reduced fat)
- Regular yogurt (low or nonfat)
- Ricotta cheese (reduced fat)
- Sour cream (reduced or nonfat)
- Soymilk
- Swiss cheese

Not Allowed:

- Any full-fat dairy products
- Butter
- Cream

Low-Glycemic Vegetables

Allowed:

- Artichoke
- Arugula
- Asparagus
- Avocado
- Bell peppers
- Broccoli
- Brussels sprouts
- Cabbage
- Cauliflower
- Celery
- Collard greens
- Cucumbers
- Eggplant
- Green beans
- Kale
- Lettuce, preferably romaine or dark leafy varieties
- Mushrooms
- Mustard greens
- Onions
- Radishes
- Spinach
- Sprouts
- Snow peas

- Summer squash
- Swiss chard
- Turnip greens
- Zucchini

High-Glycemic Vegetables

Allowed:

- Acorn squash
- Butternut squash
- Carrots
- Chickpeas
- English peas
- Spaghetti squash
- Sweet potatoes
- Tomatoes

Very Limited Quantities Allowed (One serving per week):

- Corn
- White potatoes

Low-Glycemic Fruits

Allowed:

- Bananas
- Blackberries
- Blueberries
- Cantaloupe
- Casaba melon
- Cranberries
- Grapes

- Guava
- Honeydew melon
- Lemons
- Limes
- Nectarines
- Papaya
- Peaches
- Raspberries
- Rhubarb
- Strawberries
- Watermelon

High-Glycemic Fruits

Allowed:

- Cherries
- Figs
- Grapefruit
- Kiwi
- Mango
- Oranges
- Pears
- Pineapples
- Plums
- Tangerines
- Watermelon

Fats

Allowed:

- Almonds
- Black walnuts

- Brazil nuts
- Canola oil
- Margarine or butter substitute
- Mayonnaise (low fat)
- Olive oil
- Olives (low sodium)
- Sesame seeds
- Sunflower seeds

Not Allowed:

- All other vegetable oils
- Peanut oil
- Sesame oil

Grains

Allowed:

- Almond flour
- Coconut flour
- Couscous
- Brown rice
- Wheat germ
- Whole-grain, low-carb, cold cereal
- Whole-grain, mixed-grain hot cereal
- Whole-grain, steel-cut oats
- Whole-grain bread, preferably very dense
- Whole-grain pita
- Whole-grain, thin-style bagels
- Whole-grain, thin-style English muffins
- Whole-grain tortillas
- Whole-wheat flour

Not Allowed:

- Corn meal
- Corn muffins or corn bread
- Instant or flavored oatmeal
- Sweetened cold cereals

Condiments, Seasonings, and Miscellaneous

Allowed:

- Almond butter
- Balsamic vinegar
- Caesar dressing
- Cider vinegar
- Coffee
- Dressings (no or low sodium)
- Flax seed and flax seed oil
- Herbs and spices
- Honey
- Hot sauce
- Iced tea
- Mustard (except honey mustard)
- Peanut butter (in limited quantities)
- Preserves and jellies (no or low sugar)
- Psyllium husk
- Salsa
- Sesame butter (tahini)
- Sour or dill pickles
- Soy sauce (low sodium)
- Tea
- Teriyaki sauce (low sodium)
- Tomato or spaghetti sauce (no sugar added)

- Vegetable, chicken, or beef broth (no or low sodium)
- Vinaigrette
- Whey or soy protein powder (no sugar added)

Not Allowed:

- Mayonnaise (full fat)
- Prepared Alfredo or cheese sauce
- Prepared gravy
- Regular, commercial salad dressings
- Regular sodium steak, barbecue, and other sauces

Sweets

Allowed:

- 1-ounce dark chocolate
- Dried fruits (preferably no sugar added)
- Fudge pops (fat free)
- Frozen fruit bar (no sugar added)
- Gelatin
- Ice cream (low fat)
- Popsicles
- Pudding or pudding cups (fat free)
- Sorbet or sherbet

The DASH Diet Shopping Guide

When you are on a diet, grocery shopping can be a challenging task. Here are a few tips to help make your grocery shopping easier and more nutritious.

- Buy the majority of your foods from the fresh-food sections, which are normally located around the edges of the store.

- Stay out of the aisles where processed snacks, such as chips and cookies, are located. Remember: out of sight, out of mind.
- Read the labels. Make note of the best brands so you can eventually shop without having to do any heavy reading.
- To ensure a high intake of antioxidants and micronutrients, choose different kinds of produce every time you shop. Choose lots of dark, leafy greens. Buy fruits that are rich in color, such as watermelon, mango, and dark berries. Consuming a diverse variety of produce will help increase each bite's nutritional value.
- Whenever possible, buy organic, grass-fed, or pasture-raised meats and wild seafood. Always choose the leanest cuts of whatever you're buying, and trim visible fat after cooking.
- Low-fat dairy products should be chosen whenever possible. Cheeses should be nonfat or partially nonfat. Milk should be nonfat or 1 percent fat. Yogurt should be nonfat and low in sugar or sugar free.

SECTION TWO

The DASH Diet Recipes

BREAKFASTS

Apple and Tahini Toast

Tahini is a paste made from sesame seeds, and is high in vitamins B1, B2, B3, B5, and B15. Similar to peanut butter, it's often found in dips, such as hummus. In some countries, it is commonly served for breakfast with toast.

- 2 tablespoons tahini
- 2 slices whole-wheat bread, toasted
- 1 small apple of your choice, cored and thinly sliced
- 1 teaspoon honey

Spread the tahini on the toasted bread.

Lay the apples on the bread and drizzle with honey.

Serve immediately.

Serves 1.

Breakfast Hash

Hash is a combination of meat and vegetables fried in a skillet, and is a great use of leftovers. In a healthful twist, this recipe uses an apple instead of the traditional potato.

- 2 teaspoons canola oil
- 1/4 cup onion, chopped
- 1 cup cooked turkey or chicken, chopped
- 1 tart apple, cored and chopped
- 1/2 teaspoon dried sage
- Salt substitute and freshly ground pepper, to taste
- 2 eggs
- 1 tablespoon fresh parsley, chopped

Heat a large nonstick skillet and add oil. Add onion and cook until translucent.

In a large bowl, mix the meat, apple, sage, salt substitute, and pepper. Add to onion and stir well.

Cook until meat is heated through and apple has softened.

Make 2 wells in the hash with the back of a spoon, and carefully crack in the eggs.

Cover and cook until whites are firm and yolks have cooked to desired consistency. Garnish with parsley.

Serves 2.

Crunchy Granola

Double or triple this recipe, and store leftovers in the refrigerator, where it will keep for about a week and a half. If you don't have time to squeeze your own orange juice, use store-bought juice with the pulp.

- 2 tablespoons canola oil
- 1/4 cup freshly squeezed orange juice
- 1/4 cup honey
- 1 cup oats
- 1 cup raw almonds
- 1 cup raw walnuts
- 1/4 cup sesame seeds
- 1/4 cup flax seeds
- 1 teaspoon ground cinnamon
- 1/2 teaspoon nutmeg
- 1/2 teaspoon powdered ginger
- 1/2 teaspoon salt substitute
- 1 tablespoon orange zest

Preheat oven to 350 degrees.

In a small bowl, mix the oil, orange juice, and honey together.

In a large bowl, mix together the remaining ingredients until well combined.

Drizzle the oil mixture over the dry ingredients, and stir until evenly coated.

Pack the mixture tightly into a 9 x 13–inch glass baking dish, and bake for 30 minutes until golden brown.

Let cool completely, then break into chunks and store in an airtight container.

Serve with hot or cold low-fat milk or almond milk as a cereal.

Serves 4.

Eggs Benedict

While this might not be the traditional version of eggs Benedict, you'll love this grain-free style that is as good for you as it tastes. Once you try it, you'll never want to go back to the old variety!

- 1/2 medium avocado
- 2 tablespoons lemon juice
- 1 clove garlic
- 1 large egg
- 1 tomato slice
- 2 thin slices turkey breast
- Freshly ground pepper, to taste

Put the avocado, lemon juice, and garlic in a food processor and process until smooth and creamy.

Poach the egg in a pot of simmering water until done, about 4 minutes.

To serve, place the egg on top of the tomato slice, and top with the avocado sauce and turkey.

Season with freshly ground pepper to taste.

Serves 1.

French Toast

French toast is a great breakfast dish to serve on weekends or for company. Don't forget to leave the whole-grain bread out overnight. Serve with jelly, jam, or real maple syrup.

- 1 egg
- 1/2 cup nonfat or low-fat milk
- 1/2 teaspoon pure vanilla extract
- 1/2 teaspoon cinnamon
- 4 teaspoons margarine, divided
- 4 slices whole-grain bread, cut in half

Beat egg, milk, vanilla, and cinnamon in shallow bowl until frothy.

Heat a nonstick skillet and add 1 teaspoon margarine.

Dip 2 half slices of bread into the egg mixture. Add bread to skillet and cook, turning once when the bottoms begin to brown.

When both sides are browned, transfer to a plate.

Repeat dipping and cooking the French toast, melting another teaspoon of margarine between batches until all slices are cooked.

Serves 4.

Morning Burritos

Head south of the border with this filling and tasty morning treat. If you want to turn up the heat, serve with medium or hot salsa.

- 1 teaspoon canola oil
- 4 eggs, beaten
- 2 tablespoons green chilies, chopped
- 1 cup grated, low-fat cheddar cheese, divided
- 1 cup canned black beans, rinsed and drained
- 1/2 cup mild salsa
- 4 whole-grain tortillas

Heat oil in nonstick skillet and add the eggs.

Stir in chilies and cook until the eggs are almost set.

Add 1/2 cup cheese and transfer eggs to a plate to keep warm.

Put beans and salsa into skillet, mashing the beans as they heat through.

Lay the tortillas out on a work surface.

Fill each tortilla with eggs, beans, and remaining cheese.

Top with salsa and roll up to serve.

Serves 4.

Peach and Walnut Breakfast Salad

This inspired dish is light and fresh but feels just a little bit like dessert. If you prefer, substitute apples for the peaches.

- 1/2 cup low-fat or nonfat cottage cheese, room temperature
- 1 ripe peach, pitted and sliced
- 1/4 cup chopped walnuts, toasted
- 1 teaspoon honey
- 1 tablespoon chopped fresh mint
- Zest of 1 lemon

Put the cottage cheese in a small bowl and top with the peach slices and walnuts.

Drizzle with the honey, then top with the fresh mint and a pinch of lemon zest.

Serve with a spoon.

Serves 1.

Savory Breakfast Oats

This savory hot cereal combines the fiber of oats with juicy, sunny flavors. Meanwhile, the herbs and pepper add a little zip.

- 1/2 cup steel-cut oats
- 1 cup water
- 1 large tomato, chopped
- 1 medium cucumber, chopped
- 1 tablespoon olive oil
- Fresh chopped parsley or mint for garnish
- Salt substitute and freshly ground pepper, to taste

Put the oats and 1 cup of water in a medium saucepan and bring to a boil on high heat.

Stir continuously until water is absorbed, about 15 minutes.

To serve, divide the oatmeal between 2 bowls and top with the tomatoes and cucumber.

Drizzle with olive oil, then top with the herbs.

Season to taste.

Serve immediately.

Serves 2.

Spanish Tuna Tortilla with Roasted Peppers

This recipe includes potatoes, which you are permitted to eat one serving a week.

- 6 large eggs
- 1/4 cup olive oil
- 2 small Russet potatoes, diced
- 1 small onion, chopped
- 1 roasted red bell pepper, sliced
- 1 (7-ounce) can tuna packed in water, drained well and flaked
- 2 plum tomatoes, seeded and diced
- 1 teaspoon dried tarragon

Preheat the broiler on high.

Crack the eggs in a large bowl and whisk them together until just combined.

Heat the olive oil in a large, oven-safe, nonstick or cast-iron skillet over medium-low heat.

Add the potatoes and cook until slightly soft, about 7 minutes.

Add the onion and the pepper and cook until soft, 3–5 minutes.

Add the tuna, tomatoes, and tarragon to the skillet and stir to combine, then add the eggs.

Cook for 7–10 minutes until the eggs are bubbling from the bottom and the bottom is slightly brown.

Place the skillet into the oven on 1 of the first 2 racks, and cook until the middle is set and the top is slightly brown.

Slice into wedges and serve warm or at room temperature.

Serves 4.

Spiced Scrambled Eggs

You can enjoy up to four whole eggs on the DASH diet per week. This dish uses one egg per serving, and spicy additions like the Fresno or jalapeño peppers included here not only add flavor but can help you feel full faster. Enjoy with sliced tomatoes.

- 2 tablespoons olive oil
- 1 small red onion, chopped
- 1 medium green pepper, cored, seeded, and finely chopped
- 1 red Fresno or jalapeño chili pepper, seeded and cut into thin strips
- 3 medium tomatoes, chopped
- Salt substitute and freshly ground pepper, to taste
- 1 tablespoon ground cumin
- 1 teaspoon ground coriander
- 4 large eggs, lightly beaten

Heat the olive oil in a large, heavy skillet over medium heat.

Add the onion and cook until soft and translucent, 6–7 minutes.

Add the peppers and continue to cook until soft, another 4–5 minutes.

Add in the tomatoes and season to taste.

Stir in the cumin and coriander.

Simmer for 10 minutes over medium-low heat.

Add the eggs, stirring them into the mixture to distribute.

Cover the skillet and cook until the eggs are set but still fluffy and tender, about 5–6 minutes more.

Divide between 4 plates and serve immediately.

Serves 4.

Winter Fruit Compote

A winter fruit compote uses reconstituted dried fruit and needs to be prepared in advance for breakfast. Always a smart choice for your morning meal, fruit helps supply fiber that is usually found in grains in conventional diets. Serve compote hot over cereal.

• 1/2 cup pitted prunes	• 1/2 teaspoon cinnamon
• 1/2 cup dried apples	• 1/4 teaspoon powdered ginger
• 1/2 cup dried cherries	• Pinch salt substitute

Place the fruit, spices, and salt substitute in a saucepan and cover with water.

Bring to a boil over medium heat.

Reduce heat and simmer for 5 minutes.

Turn off the heat and allow the fruit to absorb the liquid for 2 hours, or until fruit is plump.

Serves 4.

SALADS

Arugula and Artichokes

Arugula, also known as rocket, is a dark leafy green that has a peppery bite. It's very flavorful and has plenty of vitamins A, C, and K, as well as vital phytonutrients. Make this salad with the sweetest cherry tomatoes you can find.

- 4 tablespoons olive oil
- 2 tablespoons balsamic vinegar
- 1 teaspoon Dijon mustard
- 1 clove minced garlic
- 6 cups baby arugula leaves
- 6 oil-packed artichoke hearts, sliced
- 6 low-salt olives, pitted and chopped
- 1 cup cherry tomatoes, sliced in half
- 4 fresh basil leaves, thinly sliced

Make the dressing by whisking together the oil, vinegar, Dijon, and garlic until you have a smooth emulsion. Set aside.

Toss the arugula, artichokes, olives, and tomatoes together.

Drizzle the salad with the dressing, garnish with the fresh basil, and serve.

Serves 6.

Asparagus Salad

Asparagus is a spring vegetable that is as delicious raw as it is cooked. Asparagus is not only low in calories but a good source of vitamin B6, calcium, magnesium, and zinc. When choosing extra-virgin olive oil for this salad, use the highest quality available.

- 1 pound fresh asparagus
- Salt substitute and freshly ground pepper, to taste
- 4 tablespoons olive oil
- 1 tablespoon balsamic vinegar
- 1 tablespoon lemon zest

Either roast the asparagus or, with a vegetable peeler, shave it into thin strips.

Season to taste.

Toss with the oil and vinegar, garnish with a sprinkle of lemon zest, and serve.

Serves 4.

Crunchy Chicken Salad

This Asian-inspired salad is hearty, with chicken and healthful vegetables, and can be served for either lunch or dinner.

- 2 cups baby salad greens
- 1 cup broccoli florets, blanched and rinsed in cold water
- 1 cup cauliflower florets, blanched and rinsed in cold water
- 1/2 cup fresh snow peas, trimmed
- 1/2 red onion, sliced thin
- 1/4 cup low-sodium soy sauce
- 1 tablespoon cider vinegar
- 1 tablespoon olive oil
- 1 teaspoon honey
- 1 teaspoon sesame seeds, toasted
- 1 cup cooked chicken, cubed

Toss greens, broccoli, cauliflower, snow peas, and onion in large bowl.

Whisk soy sauce, vinegar, olive oil, honey, and sesame seeds in a small bowl, and pour over greens.

Toss salad and transfer to plates.

Top each portion with chicken.

Serves 4.

Four-Bean Salad

High in fiber, beans are also versatile and can be eaten hot or cold, in salads or soups. Use dried beans for the best flavor, but keep canned beans on hand as a convenient option—just be sure to read the labels for hidden salt.

- 1/2 cup white beans, cooked
- 1/2 cup black-eyed peas, cooked
- 1/2 cup fava beans, cooked
- 1/2 cup lima beans, cooked
- 1 red bell pepper, diced
- 1 small bunch parsley, chopped
- 2 tablespoons olive oil
- 1 teaspoon ground cumin
- Juice of 1 lemon
- Salt substitute and freshly ground pepper, to taste

You can cook the beans a day or two in advance to speed up the preparation of this dish.

Combine all ingredients in a large bowl and mix well.

Season to taste.

Allow to sit for 30 minutes, so the flavors can come together before serving.

Serves 4.

Double-Apple Spinach Salad

This salad is crunchy, tart, and sweet, with greens, fruits, nuts, and low-fat cheese. Its ingredients also provide a wide range of benefits—apples, walnuts, and spinach offer plenty of fiber, vitamins, minerals, and antioxidants. Serve for lunch with a whole-grain baguette, or at dinner as a first course.

- 8 cups fresh baby spinach
- 1 medium Granny Smith apple, diced
- 1 medium red apple, diced
- 1/2 cup toasted walnuts
- 2 ounces low-fat, sharp, white cheddar cheese, cubed
- 3 tablespoons olive oil
- 1 tablespoon red wine vinegar or apple cider vinegar

Toss the spinach, apples, walnuts, and cubed cheese together.

Lightly drizzle oil and vinegar over top and serve.

Serves 4.

Garden Salad with Sardine Filets

Sardines are a super-food, adding vitamin B12, tryptophan, selenium, omega-3 fats, protein, phosphorus, vitamin D, calcium, and vitamin B3. You can serve this salad equally well as a side or a main dish.

- 1/2 cup olive oil
- Juice of 1 medium lemon
- 1 teaspoon Dijon mustard
- Salt substitute and freshly ground pepper, to taste
- 4 medium tomatoes, diced
- 1 large cucumber, peeled and diced
- 1 pound arugula, trimmed and chopped
- 1 small red onion, thinly sliced
- 1 small bunch flat-leaf parsley, chopped
- 4 whole sardine filets packed in olive oil, drained and chopped

For the dressing, whisk together the olive oil, lemon juice, and mustard, and season with salt substitute and freshly ground pepper. Set aside.

In a large bowl, combine all the vegetables with the parsley, and toss.

Add the sardine filets on top of the salad.

Drizzle the dressing over the salad just before serving.

Serves 6.

Peachy Tomato Salad

This is a super-easy, summer side dish that is perfect when both tomatoes and peaches are at their best.

- 2 ripe peaches, halved, pitted, and sliced into wedges
- 2 ripe tomatoes, cut into wedges
- 1/2 red onion, thinly sliced
- Salt substitute and freshly ground pepper, to taste
- 3 tablespoons olive oil
- 1 tablespoon lemon juice

Toss the peaches, tomatoes, and red onion in a large bowl.

Season to taste.

Add the olive oil and lemon juice, and gently toss.

Serve at room temperature.

Serves 2.

Raw Zucchini Salad

This light and robust salad makes an excellent starter. Zucchini and tomatoes are both summer vegetables that provide good nutrition as well as hydration. The key to creating this dish is to slice the zucchini paper thin or shred into long, thin slices with a cheese grater.

- 1 medium zucchini, sliced paper thin
- 6 cherry tomatoes, halved
- 3 tablespoons olive oil
- Juice of 1 lemon
- Salt substitute and freshly ground pepper, to taste
- 3–4 basil leaves, thinly sliced
- 2 tablespoons freshly grated, low-fat Parmesan cheese

Layer the zucchini slices on 2 plates in even layers.

Top with the tomatoes.

Drizzle with the olive oil and lemon juice.

Season to taste.

Top with the basil and sprinkle with cheese before serving.

Serves 2.

Riviera Tuna Salad

Humble, canned tuna becomes something special in this healthful, main-dish salad, while garbanzo beans add fiber and protein.

- 1/4 cup olive oil
- 1/4 cup balsamic vinegar
- 1/2 teaspoon minced garlic
- 1/4 teaspoon dried oregano
- Salt substitute and freshly ground pepper, to taste
- 2 tablespoons capers, drained

- 4–6 cups baby greens
- 1 (6-ounce) can solid white albacore tuna, drained
- 1 cup canned garbanzo beans, rinsed and drained
- 1/4 cup pitted, low-salt olives, quartered
- 2 Roma tomatoes, chopped

To make the vinaigrette, whisk together the oil, balsamic vinegar, garlic, oregano, salt substitute, and freshly ground pepper until emulsified.

Stir in the capers.

Refrigerate for up to 6 hours before serving.

Place the baby greens in a salad bowl or on individual plates, and top with the tuna, beans, olives, and tomatoes.

Drizzle the vinaigrette over all, and serve immediately.

Serves 4.

Wilted Kale Salad

Kale can be eaten raw, cooked, or gently sautéed—as it is in this recipe—with a little garlic, olive oil, and cherry tomatoes. A nutrient powerhouse, kale is extremely high in vitamins A, C, and K. Use a lid to help wilt the kale and keep it in the pan.

- 2 heads kale
- 1+ tablespoon olive oil
- 2 cloves garlic, minced
- 1 cup cherry tomatoes, sliced
- Salt substitute and freshly ground pepper, to taste
- Juice of 1 lemon

Rinse and dry kale.

Tear the kale into bite-sized pieces.

Heat 1 tablespoon of the olive oil in a large skillet, and add the garlic.

Cook for 1 minute and then add the kale.

Cook just until wilted, then add the tomatoes.

Cook until tomatoes are softened, then remove from heat.

Place tomatoes and kale in a bowl, and season with salt substitute and freshly ground pepper.

Drizzle with remaining olive oil and lemon juice, serve, and enjoy.

Serves 4.

SIDES AND SNACKS

Baked Kale Chips

If you're looking for a crunchy snack to munch on instead of potato chips, you'll love these kale chips. Kale is extremely low in calories and is one of the most nutrient-dense foods on the planet. Experiment with different salt substitute flavors.

- 2 heads curly leaf kale
- 2 tablespoons olive oil

- Salt substitute, to taste

Tear the kale into bite-sized pieces.

Toss with the olive oil, and lay on a baking sheet in a single layer.

Sprinkle with a pinch of salt substitute.

Bake for 10–15 minutes until crispy.

Serve or store in an airtight container.

Makes about 4 cups chips.

Chili Shrimp

This tasty and spicy side dish is great for potlucks and other fun occasions.

- 1/2 cup olive oil
- 5 cloves garlic, minced
- 1 teaspoon red pepper flakes
- 24 large fresh shrimp, peeled and deveined
- Juice of 1 lemon
- Salt substitute and freshly ground pepper, to taste

Heat the oil in a large skillet over medium-high heat.

Add the garlic and red pepper flakes, and cook for 1 minute.

Add the shrimp and cook an additional 3 minutes, stirring frequently.

Remove from the pan, and sprinkle with lemon juice and salt substitute.

Serves 6.

Classic Hummus

Hummus is a creamy and delicious dip that can be served as an appetizer, at a party, or just as a snack. Try using hummus in place of mayonnaise on sandwiches.

- 3 cups cooked chickpeas, slightly warmed
- 1/4 cup olive oil
- Juice of 2 lemons
- 2–3 cloves garlic
- 3/4 cup tahini
- Salt substitute and freshly ground pepper, to taste
- 1/2 cup pine nuts, toasted (optional)
- 1/4 cup fresh flat-leaf parsley, chopped
- Assorted fresh veggies or whole-wheat pita for dipping

Add the chickpeas, olive oil, lemon juice, and garlic to a food processor, and puree until smooth.

Add the tahini and continue to blend until creamy.

If too thick, a bit of water can be used to thin it out.

Season with salt substitute and freshly ground pepper to taste.

Add the pine nuts if desired, and garnish with chopped parsley.

Serve with fresh veggies and whole-wheat pita wedges.

Serves 6–8.

Curry Onion Dip

The curry flavor of this scrumptious dip will strengthen the longer this dip stands, so make it a day in advance.

- 1 cup raw almonds
- 1 onion, chopped
- 3 tablespoons fresh lime juice
- 3 tablespoons olive oil
- 1 teaspoon curry powder
- 1/2 teaspoon salt substitute
- 1/2 teaspoon freshly ground pepper
- 1/2 teaspoon paprika

Put all ingredients in a food processor and blend until smooth, scraping down sides as needed.

Will keep in refrigerator for up to a week.

Serves 4.

Mini Lettuce Wraps

Like a Greek salad wrapped in lettuce, this bite-sized appetizer is easy to assemble. Swap out the tomatoes, cucumbers, and/or red onion for any vegetables you like. Serve the wraps on their own or as part of a larger selection of appetizers.

- 1 tomato, diced
- 1 cucumber, diced
- 1 red onion, sliced
- 1 ounce low-fat feta cheese, crumbled
- Juice of 1 lemon
- 1 tablespoon olive oil
- Salt substitute and freshly ground pepper, to taste
- 12 small, intact iceberg lettuce leaves

Combine the tomato, cucumber, onion, and feta in a bowl with the lemon juice and olive oil.

Season with salt substitute and freshly ground pepper.

Without tearing the leaves, gently fill each leaf with a tablespoon of the veggie mixture.

Roll them as tightly as you can, and lay them seam-side-down on a serving platter.

Makes about 1 dozen wraps.

Sardines in Tomato Sauce

Sardines are plentiful, cheap, and sustainable. Best of all, they're full of healthful omega-3 fatty acids. They're easy to prepare, since the spine lifts out easily and takes all the bones with it.

- 2 pounds fresh sardines
- 3 tablespoons olive oil, divided
- 1 small onion, sliced thinly
- 4 Roma tomatoes, peeled and chopped
- Zest of 1 orange
- Salt substitute and freshly ground pepper, to taste
- 2 tablespoons whole-wheat breadcrumbs
- 1/2 cup white wine

Preheat the oven to 425 degrees.

Clean the sardines under running water.

Slit the belly, remove the spine, and butterfly the fish.

Brush a little olive oil in a baking dish.

Heat the remaining olive oil in a large skillet.

Add the onion, tomatoes, orange zest, salt substitute, and pepper, and simmer for 20 minutes, or until the mixture thickens and softens.

Place half the sauce in the bottom of the casserole dish.

Set the fish on top, and spread the remaining sauce over the fish.

Top with the breadcrumbs and white wine, and bake for 20 minutes.

Serve immediately.

Serves 4.

Savory Mixed Nuts

If you're having trouble giving up on packaged nuts, which often include preservatives, sugar, and too much salt, make this recipe for those times you're just "nuts for nuts."

- 2 cups raw nuts like almonds, walnuts, or pecans
- 1 tablespoon olive oil
- 1 teaspoon salt substitute (choose your favorite flavor)

Preheat oven to 350 degrees.

Place nuts in a bowl and drizzle with oil.

Toss until evenly coated, then sprinkle with seasoned salt substitute, and toss again.

Place in a single layer on a large baking sheet, and bake for 20 minutes.

Stir after 10 minutes.

Serves 4.

Spinach Dip

This creamy mixture uses avocado instead of sour cream, but you'll enjoy this dip too much to even notice the difference. We suggest dipping celery and carrot sticks, but try cucumber, radish, and zucchini as well.

- 1 (10-ounce) package frozen chopped spinach
- 1 ripe avocado
- 1 tablespoon fresh lemon juice
- 1 small onion, chopped
- 1 teaspoon salt substitute
- Fresh celery and carrot sticks for dipping

Cook spinach in microwave just until defrosted. Set aside to cool.

Slice avocado in half and remove pit. Scoop flesh into food processor and sprinkle with lemon juice.

Squeeze spinach until almost dry and add to processor with onion and salt substitute.

Process for 1 minute until smooth.

Keeps for up to 2 days in refrigerator.

Serves 4.

Toasted Pita Wedges

A sandwich-style pocket bread, pita can be served alongside salads and soups with dips and spreads. You can buy pita chips, but their salt content can be prohibitive. These wedges are easy to prepare and much healthier since you control the ingredients.

- 4 whole-wheat pita rounds
- 1 tablespoon olive oil
- 1 teaspoon garlic powder
- 1/4 teaspoon paprika
- Salt substitute and freshly ground pepper, to taste

Preheat oven to 400 degrees.

Cut the pita rounds into 8 wedges each, and lay on a parchment-lined baking sheet in an even layer.

Drizzle with olive oil, and sprinkle with garlic powder and paprika.

Season with salt substitute and freshly ground pepper.

Bake for 10–12 minutes, until wedges are lightly browned and crisp.

Allow to cool completely before serving for crisper wedges.

Makes 32 wedges.

Tropical Fruit and Yogurt Bowl

This combination of fruit and yogurt makes a great breakfast but can also be served as an afternoon snack. It's loaded with vitamin C, essential enzymes, and antioxidants.

- 1/2 cup fresh pineapple, diced
- 1/2 cup fresh mango, diced
- 1/2 cup fresh papaya, diced
- 1 cup low-fat unsweetened yogurt
- Fresh mint
- Optional: honey, cinnamon, or low-fat granola

Combine the fruit and yogurt in a bowl and stir gently.

Transfer to 2 individual bowls.

If desired, top each serving with a small drizzle of honey or a dash of cinnamon, or stir in a couple tablespoons of granola.

Garnish with a couple fresh mint leaves.

Serves 2.

SOUPS

Beans and Chard Soup

This simple soup is rustic and soothing yet nutritionally powerful. Serve it with a green salad and a slice of whole-grain bread.

- 1 cup dried pinto beans, soaked overnight
- 1/4 cup olive oil
- 1 medium onion, diced
- 4 cups chicken stock or water
- 2 cups chard or Swiss chard, sliced, tough stems removed
- 1 medium tomato, diced
- 1/2 teaspoon thyme
- Salt substitute and freshly ground pepper, to taste

Drain and rinse the soaked pinto beans.

Heat the olive oil in a stockpot over medium heat.

Sauté the onion for 5–8 minutes, or until tender and translucent.

Add the remaining ingredients, including the pinto beans, and heat to a simmer.

Cover and cook on low for 1–2 hours, or until the beans are tender, but not falling apart.

Season to taste with salt substitute and freshly ground pepper.

Serves 6.

Chicken Soup

Spring asparagus, peas, spinach, and chives add freshness to this chicken soup.

- 1 (32-ounce) carton chicken broth
- 1 (10-ounce) package frozen peas and pearl onions
- 1 carrot, peeled and sliced thin
- 1 bunch asparagus, trimmed and cut into 1-inch pieces
- 1 cup fresh spinach, chopped
- 1/2 teaspoon dried marjoram
- 1/2 teaspoon salt substitute
- 1/4 teaspoon freshly ground pepper
- 1/4 teaspoon ground nutmeg
- 1 cup cooked chicken, diced
- 2 tablespoons arrowroot
- 1/4 cup cold water
- 1/2 cup chives, chopped

Bring broth to a boil in a soup pot over high heat.

Add peas and carrot, and reduce heat to a simmer.

Cook for 2 minutes, and add asparagus, spinach, and seasonings.

Cook for 5 minutes, or until vegetables are tender. Increase heat and add chicken.

In small bowl, combine arrowroot with cold water, and mix until thoroughly blended.

Add to the hot soup, stirring until slightly thickened. Remove from heat and stir in chives just before serving.

Serves 4.

Cold Cucumber Soup

Nothing's more refreshing on a hot day than this classic, chilled soup. Serve it with a salad for a light lunch or dinner.

- 2 seedless cucumbers, peeled and cut into chunks
- 2 cups plain Greek yogurt
- 1/2 cup mint, finely chopped
- 2 garlic cloves, minced
- 2 cups chicken broth or vegetable stock
- 3 teaspoons fresh dill
- 1 tablespoon tomato paste
- Salt substitute and freshly ground pepper, to taste

Puree the cucumber, yogurt, mint, and garlic in a food processor or blender.

Add the chicken broth, dill, tomato paste, salt substitute, and freshly ground pepper, and blend to incorporate.

Refrigerate for at least 2 hours before serving.

Serves 4.

Lentil Soup with Spinach

Lentils are similar to beans as far as flavor and nutrients go, but they have one distinct advantage when it comes to preparation: they cook much faster. Though rich and creamy, they are also very low in calories.

- 1 teaspoon olive oil
- 1 cup onion, chopped
- 1 1/2 cups lentils
- 1 tablespoon curry powder
- 6 cups water
- 12 ounces fresh spinach

Heat the olive oil and sauté the onion.

Add the lentils and curry powder and stir.

Add the water and cook until lentils are tender, about 15–20 minutes.

Add the spinach and stir until wilted.

Serve with toasted whole-wheat bread and a green salad.

Serves 6.

Roasted Eggplant Soup

Fresh herbs add flavor to this soup as well as powerful nutrients and antioxidants. This makes an excellent meal on its own if served with bread, but it can also be served as a first course.

- 3 large eggplants, sliced lengthwise
- Pinch salt substitute
- 2 tablespoons olive oil
- 1 medium red onion, chopped
- 2 tablespoons garlic, minced
- 1 teaspoon dried thyme
- Salt substitute and freshly ground pepper, to taste
- 2 large, ripe tomatoes, halved
- 5 cups chicken broth
- 1/4 cup low-fat cream
- Small bunch fresh mint, chopped

Preheat oven to 400 degrees.

"Salt" both sides of the sliced eggplant, and let sit for 20 minutes to draw out the bitter juices.

Rinse the eggplant and pat dry with a paper towel.

Place the eggplants on a sheet pan, and put them in the oven.

Roast for 45 minutes. Remove from oven and allow to cool.

When cool, remove all of the insides, discarding the skins.

Heat the oil in a large skillet over medium heat.

Add the onions and garlic, and cook for 5 minutes until soft and translucent.

Add the thyme and season with salt substitute and freshly ground pepper.

Put the eggplant, tomatoes, and onion in a food processor, and process until smooth.

Put the chicken broth in a pot, and bring to a boil. Reduce heat to a simmer, and add the eggplant mixture.

Stir until well combined, and fold in the cream.

Season to taste.

Serve the soup garnished with the fresh mint.

Serves 8.

Spinach and Brown Rice Soup

This recipe calls for a lot of spinach; however, cooking the spinach reduces its volume significantly.

- 1 tablespoon olive oil
- 1 large onion, chopped
- 2 cloves garlic, minced
- 3 pounds fresh spinach leaves, stems removed and leaves chopped

- 8 cups chicken broth
- 1/2 cup long-grain brown rice
- Salt substitute and freshly ground pepper, to taste

Heat the olive oil in a large Dutch oven over medium heat, and add the onion and garlic.

Cook until the onion are soft and translucent, about 5 minutes.

Add the spinach and stir.

Cover the pot and cook the spinach until wilted, about 3 more minutes.

Using a slotted spoon, remove the spinach and onion from the pot, leaving the liquid.

Put the spinach mixture in a food processor or blender and process until smooth, then return to the pot.

Add the chicken broth and bring to a boil.

Add the rice, reduce heat, and simmer until rice is cooked, about 45 minutes.

Season to taste.

Serve hot.

Serves 6.

Tomato Soup

This version of tomato soup is subtly flavored with the classic spices of Morocco—paprika, ginger, cumin, and cinnamon. In terms of nutrients, cooked tomatoes are a great source of lycopene.

- 2 tablespoons olive oil
- 1 large onion, coarsely chopped
- 8 large tomatoes, seeded and coarsely chopped
- 1 teaspoon paprika
- 1 teaspoon fresh ginger, finely chopped
- 1 teaspoon ground cumin
- 2 cups chicken broth
- 1 cinnamon stick
- 1 teaspoon honey
- Salt substitute and freshly ground pepper, to taste
- Juice of 1 lemon
- 1 small bunch parsley, chopped
- 2 tablespoons chopped cilantro

Heat a large Dutch oven over medium-high heat.

Add the olive oil and onion, and cook until soft and translucent.

Add the tomatoes and the seasonings and stir.

Pour in the chicken broth, and add the cinnamon stick and honey.

Simmer for 15 minutes, then puree the soup in a food processor or blender (remove the cinnamon stick for this step and return it when done).

Pour back into the pot, and season with salt substitute and freshly ground pepper to taste.

Stir in the lemon juice and serve garnished with the parsley and cilantro.

Serves 6.

Turkish Lentil Soup

Lentil soup is one of the most inexpensive, nutritious foods you can make. If you can't find green lentils, substitute brown. This Turkish-inspired recipe is vegetarian, but feel free to add shredded chicken for a more robust dish.

- 2 tablespoons olive oil
- 1 small onion, diced
- 2 tablespoons flour
- 4 cups water or chicken stock
- 1 1/2 cups green lentils
- 1 carrot, peeled and diced
- 1/2 teaspoon dried thyme
- 1 teaspoon salt substitute
- 1/2 teaspoon freshly ground pepper

Heat the olive oil in a large stockpot on medium-high heat.

Sauté the onion just until tender and translucent.

Whisk in the flour, stirring for 30 seconds until thickened into a paste.

Slowly, whisk in the water or chicken stock 1/4 cup at a time, and bring to a boil, stirring frequently.

Add the lentils, carrot, and seasonings. Cover and simmer for 1 hour, or until lentils are tender.

Serves 6.

White Bean, Cherry Tomato, and Kale Soup

This soup is as inexpensive as it is filling and nutritious. If you want to make this completely vegetarian, substitute vegetable broth for chicken.

- 2 tablespoons olive oil
- 1 small onion, chopped
- 2 cloves garlic, minced
- 1 bunch kale, torn into bite-sized pieces
- 6 cups chicken or vegetable broth
- 2 pints cherry tomatoes, halved
- 2 cans white beans of your choice, drained and rinsed
- Salt substitute and freshly ground pepper, to taste
- Freshly grated, low-fat Parmesan cheese

Heat the oil in a large soup pot or Dutch oven over medium heat.

Add the onion and cook for 5 minutes, or until soft and translucent.

Add the garlic and cook for 1 more minute.

Add the kale and stir until well coated with the oil.

Add the broth and bring to boil on high heat.

Reduce heat to low, and simmer for 15 minutes, until kale is softened.

Add the tomatoes and beans, and simmer for 5 more minutes.

Season with salt substitute and freshly ground pepper to taste.

To serve, ladle into bowls, and sprinkle with freshly grated, low-fat Parmesan cheese.

Serves 4.

Zuppa di Fagioli

Traditionally, this Tuscan soup is made with cannellini beans or cranberry beans, and the locals are known as "bean eaters." Nutritionally, beans are great for lowering cholesterol. If you can't find cannellini beans, use navy beans, white beans, or even chickpeas.

- 2 tablespoons olive oil
- 3 carrots, peeled and diced
- 1 onion, chopped
- 2 cloves garlic, chopped
- 8 cups water or chicken broth
- 2 cups dried beans, soaked overnight, rinsed and drained
- 1 teaspoon fresh thyme
- 1 bay leaf
- Salt substitute and freshly ground pepper, to taste
- 8 slices whole-wheat bread
- Low-fat Parmesan cheese

Heat the olive oil in a large stockpot on medium heat.

Add the carrots and onion, and sauté until the onion is translucent.

Add the garlic and sauté 1 minute more.

Add the water or chicken broth, the beans, and the seasonings, and cover.

Bring to a boil on high heat, then reduce heat and simmer for 2 hours, or until the beans are tender.

Season to taste and top with a slice of toasted whole-wheat bread and grated Parmesan cheese.

Serves 8.

SANDWICHES AND WRAPS

Avocado and Asparagus Wraps

Avocados are not just for guacamole—they provide a great addition to your diet because of their healthful fats. Use mashed avocados in place of mayonnaise in salads, sandwiches, and wraps. This wrap is served warm, and can also work as a light meal or snack.

- 12 spears asparagus
- 1 ripe avocado, mashed slightly
- Juice of 1 lime
- 2 cloves garlic, minced
- 2 cups brown rice, cooked and chilled
- 3 tablespoons Greek yogurt
- Salt substitute and freshly ground pepper, to taste
- 3 (8-inch) whole-grain tortillas
- 1/2 cup cilantro, diced
- 2 tablespoons red onion, diced

Steam asparagus in microwave or stove top steamer until tender.

Mash the avocado, lime juice, and garlic in a medium-mixing bowl.

In a separate bowl, mix the rice and yogurt.

Season both mixtures with salt substitute and freshly ground pepper to taste.

Heat the tortillas in a dry nonstick skillet.

Spread each tortilla with the avocado mixture, and top with the rice, cilantro, and onion, followed by the asparagus.

Fold up both sides of the tortilla, and roll tightly to close. Cut in half diagonally before serving.

Serves 6.

Avocado Cheese Melt

Mashed avocado can sometimes be a good substitute for butter. It adds richness to this creative twist on a grilled cheese sandwich.

- 1 ripe avocado, peeled and pitted
- 4 slices whole-grain bread
- 4 ounces thin-sliced Swiss cheese

Mash half the avocado in a bowl, and slice the other half thinly.

Spread the mashed avocado on the bread slices, and top each with a slice of cheese.

Arrange the sliced avocado on top of the cheese.

Broil for several minutes, until the cheese is melted.

Serves 4.

Creamy Seafood Salad

This salad is great on its own or as a sandwich filling. Serve with low-sodium crackers or a bowl of soup.

- 6 ounces fresh, cooked crab or low-sodium artificial crab
- 4 ounces fresh, cooked bay shrimp
- 2 green onions, diced
- 1/2 cup celery, finely chopped
- 1/2 cup fresh grapefruit, finely chopped
- 1/4 cup low-sodium Italian salad dressing
- 1/4 cup fat-free sour cream
- 1/4 teaspoon ground cardamom
- 1 teaspoon fresh cilantro, chopped
- Head of romaine lettuce or 8 slices whole-wheat bread

Combine all ingredients, with the exception of the romaine, in a salad bowl and chill.

Serve on a bed of romaine lettuce or make sandwiches.

Serves 4.

Cucumber Basil Sandwiches

The addition of basil adds antioxidants and flavor to this hummus sandwich. The skin and seeds of the cucumber contain many nutrients, so don't remove them. If you like, make it an open-faced sandwich to further reduce the carbohydrates and calories.

• 4 slices whole-grain bread   • 1 large cucumber, thinly sliced

• 1/4 cup hummus   • 4 whole basil leaves

Spread the hummus on 2 slices of bread, and layer the cucumbers onto it.

Top with the basil leaves and close the sandwiches.

Press down lightly and serve immediately.

Serves 2.

Grilled Chicken Salad Wrap

Tender and juicy grilled chicken, topped with fresh vegetables, and wrapped in a whole-grain tortilla makes a filling and hearty meal. Serve this with celery and carrot sticks on the side for crunch instead of salty chips.

- 1 boneless, skinless chicken breast
- Salt substitute and freshly ground pepper, to taste
- 1 cup baby spinach
- 1 roasted red pepper, sliced
- 1 tomato, chopped
- 1/2 small red onion, thinly sliced
- 1/2 small cucumber, chopped
- 4 tablespoons olive oil
- Juice of 1 lemon
- 1 whole-wheat tortilla

Preheat a gas or charcoal grill to medium-high heat.

Season the chicken breast with salt substitute and freshly ground pepper, and grill until cooked through, about 7–8 minutes per side.

Allow chicken to rest for 5 minutes before slicing into strips.

While the chicken is cooking, put all the vegetables into a medium-sized mixing bowl and season with salt substitute and freshly ground pepper.

Chop the chicken into cubes and add to salad.

Add the olive oil and lemon juice and toss well.

Place the mixture onto a tortilla and wrap.

Serve immediately.

Serves 1.

Mediterranean Tuna Salad Sandwiches

Usually loaded with high-fat mayonnaise, tuna salad does not often come to mind as a healthful staple. This version is made with Greek yogurt and flavorful roasted peppers, adding taste and moisture without a lot of fat. You can also enjoy the tuna salad without the bread, if you prefer.

- 1 can white tuna, packed in water or olive oil
- 1 roasted red pepper, diced
- 1/2 small red onion, diced
- 10 low-salt olives, finely chopped
- 1/4 cup plain Greek yogurt
- 1 tablespoon fresh parsley, chopped
- Juice of 1 lemon
- Salt substitute and freshly ground pepper, to taste
- 4 whole-grain pieces of bread

In a small bowl, combine all of the ingredients except the bread, and mix well.

Season with salt substitute and freshly ground pepper to taste.

Toast the bread or warm in a pan.

Make the sandwich and serve immediately.

Serves 2.

New York Turkey Melt

This recipe will help you satisfy the urge for a deli sandwich. A variety of vegetables and cheeses add to the texture and flavor of this deluxe hero.

- 4 slices low-sodium rye bread or whole-wheat flatbread
- 2 tablespoons fat-free cream cheese
- 1 teaspoon prepared horseradish
- 6 ounces sliced, homemade, roast turkey breast
- 1/2 small cucumber, very thinly sliced
- 1/2 small red onion, very thinly sliced
- 2 thin slices provolone
- Canola oil spray

Spread 2 of the bread slices with cream cheese and horseradish, and then layer on the turkey, cucumber, onion, and provolone.

Top each with another slice of bread.

Coat a nonstick skillet lightly with canola oil spray, and toast the sandwiches over medium heat until well browned.

Serves 2.

Open-Faced Eggplant Parmesan Sandwich

Eggplant Parmesan is often deep fried, laden with high-fat cheese, and served with mounds of pasta. In this version, the eggplant is broiled before being topped with marinara and low-fat Parmesan cheese, and served on a slice of toasted whole-grain bread. Eat with a knife and fork!

- 1 small eggplant, sliced into 1/4-inch rounds
- Pinch salt substitute
- 2 tablespoons olive oil
- Salt substitute and freshly ground pepper, to taste
- 2 slices whole-grain bread, thickly cut and toasted
- 1 cup marinara sauce (no added sugar)
- 1/4 cup freshly grated, low-fat Parmesan cheese

Preheat broiler to high heat.

"Salt" both sides of the sliced eggplant, and let sit for 20 minutes to draw out the bitter juices.

Rinse the eggplant and pat dry with a paper towel.

Brush the eggplant with the olive oil, and season with salt substitute and freshly ground pepper.

Lay the eggplant on a sheet pan, and broil until crisp, about 4 minutes.

Flip over and crisp the other side.

Lay the toasted bread on a sheet pan.

Spoon some marinara sauce on each slice of bread, and layer the eggplant on top.

Sprinkle half of the cheese on top of the eggplant and top with more marinara sauce.

Sprinkle with remaining cheese.

Put the sandwiches under the broiler until the cheese has melted, about 2 minutes.

Using a spatula, transfer the sandwiches to plates and serve.

Serves 2.

Slow-Roasted Tomato and Basil Panini

Slow-roasting tomatoes brings out their flavor, and cooking them actually increases their lycopene. Here the flavors of an Italian Caprese salad are transformed into a sandwich. If you don't have a panini maker or grill pan, you can easily toast the sandwich in a nonstick skillet.

- 4 Roma tomatoes, halved
- 4 cloves garlic
- 2 tablespoons olive oil
- 1 tablespoon Italian seasoning
- Salt substitute and freshly ground pepper, to taste
- 4 basil leaves
- 2 slices fresh mozzarella
- 4 slices whole-grain bread

Preheat oven to 250 degrees.

Lay the tomatoes and garlic cloves on a sheet pan, and drizzle with the olive oil.

Sprinkle with Italian seasoning, and season with salt substitute and freshly ground pepper.

Roast for about 2 1/2–3 hours, until tomatoes are extremely fragrant and slightly wilted.

To make your panini, layer the tomatoes with the basil and cheese on the bread.

Preheat a panini maker, and cook the sandwiches until the bread is browned and the cheese is melted.

Place another pan on top to press the sandwich.

Flip the panini after 3–4 minutes when the bread has nice grill marks, and cook the other side.

Serve warm.

Serves 2.

Spinach and Mushroom Pita

This easy-to-put-together pita pocket makes a light and healthful lunch option. All of the ingredients in the sandwich can also be used in salads, so stock up your refrigerator produce drawer!

- 2 cups baby spinach leaves
- 1 small red onion, thinly sliced
- 1/2 cup button mushrooms, sliced
- 1/2 cup alfalfa sprouts
- 1 tomato, chopped
- 1/2 small cucumber
- 2 tablespoons olive oil
- Juice of 1 lemon
- Salt substitute and freshly ground pepper, to taste
- 2 whole-grain pita pockets

Combine all the vegetables, mushrooms, olive oil, and lemon juice in a bowl, and season with salt substitute and freshly ground pepper to taste.

Toss the salad until well mixed.

Stuff the vegetable mixture into the pita pockets and serve immediately.

Serves 2.

Turkey Leftover Sandwich

This recipe is great, especially when you're craving Thanksgiving leftovers. Take it for lunch or prepare it for a quick weekend dinner.

- 1 whole-wheat hoagie roll
- 1 tablespoon nonfat cream cheese
- 1 teaspoon Dijon mustard
- 1/2 teaspoon prepared horseradish
- 4 ounces homemade or low-salt deli turkey breast, thinly sliced
- 2 tablespoons whole-berry cranberry sauce
- 1 ounce Swiss cheese, thinly sliced
- 1 cup fresh alfalfa sprouts

Spread 1/2 of the hoagie roll with the cream cheese and the other half with the mustard and horseradish combined.

Layer the turkey onto the roll with the cranberry sauce, Swiss cheese, and sprouts.

Serve with a salad or cup of low-sodium soup.

Serves 1.

GRAINS AND PASTAS

Baked Ziti

Baked ziti is an American classic and the perfect dish for potlucks. Using whole-wheat pasta, low-fat cheeses, and homemade marinara sauce makes it healthier and lighter, but watch your portion size, since there's still a lot of dairy.

For the marinara sauce:

- 2 tablespoons olive oil
- 1/4 medium onion, diced (about 3 tablespoons)
- 3 cloves garlic, chopped
- 1 (28-ounce) can whole, peeled tomatoes, roughly chopped
- Sprig of fresh thyme
- 1/2 bunch fresh basil
- Salt substitute and freshly ground pepper, to taste

For the ziti:

- 1 pound whole-wheat ziti
- 3 1/2 cups marinara sauce, divided
- 1 cup low-fat cottage cheese
- 1 cup grated, low-fat mozzarella cheese, divided
- 3/4 cup freshly grated Parmesan cheese

Marinara Sauce:

Heat the oil in a medium saucepan over medium-high heat.

Sauté the onion and garlic, stirring, until lightly browned, about 3 minutes.

Add the tomatoes and the herbs, and bring to a boil.

Lower the heat and simmer, covered, for 10 minutes.

Remove and discard the herb sprigs.

Stir in salt substitute and season with freshly ground pepper to taste.

Ziti:

Preheat the oven to 375 degrees.

Prepare the pasta according to package directions.

Drain pasta.

Combine the pasta in a bowl with 2 cups marinara sauce, the cottage cheese, and half the mozzarella and Parmesan cheeses.

Spread the mixture in a baking dish, and top with the remaining marinara sauce and cheese.

Bake for 30–40 minutes, or until bubbly and golden brown.

Serves 8.

Brown Rice with Apricots, Cherries, and Toasted Pecans

Brown rice is a great source of fiber and combines easily with lots of other healthful additions. The dried apricots and cherries add tartness to this dish, while the pecans add crunch and extra flavor. If you prefer, use walnuts or almonds in place of the pecans.

- 2 tablespoons olive oil
- 2 green onions, sliced
- 1/2 cup brown rice
- 1 cup chicken stock
- 4–5 dried apricots, chopped
- 2 tablespoons dried cherries
- 2 tablespoons pecans, toasted and chopped
- Salt substitute and freshly ground pepper, to taste

Heat the oil in a medium saucepan, and add the green onions.

Sauté for 1–2 minutes, then add the rice. Stir to coat in oil, then add the stock.

Bring to a boil, reduce heat, and cover.

Simmer for 50 minutes.

Remove lid, add the apricots, cherries, and pecans, and cover for 10 more minutes.

Fluff with a fork to mix the fruit into the rice, season with salt substitute and freshly ground pepper, and serve.

Serves 2.

Cumin-Scented Lentils with Rice

This classic Lebanese dish, called Megadarra, pairs well with chicken or fish.

- 1/4 cup olive oil
- 1 medium onion, thinly sliced
- 1 tablespoon ground cumin
- 1 cup green lentils
- 2 cups water divided

- 3/4 cup long-grain brown rice, rinsed
- 2 bay leaves
- Salt substitute and freshly ground pepper, to taste

Heat a large saucepan over medium heat.

Add the olive oil and onion, and sauté for 10 minutes until soft and translucent.

Add the cumin and stir to incorporate.

Add the lentils and stir to coat in the oil.

Add 1 cup water, bring to a boil, and reduce to a simmer.

Simmer for 15 minutes, until most of the water has been absorbed.

Add the rice to the pot, along with another cup of water and the bay leaves, and bring to a boil.

Reduce heat, cover, and simmer for 15–20 more minutes, checking periodically and adding water to prevent rice or lentils from becoming scorched.

When both the rice and lentils are tender and cooked through, stir and season with salt substitute and freshly ground pepper.

Remove the bay leaves and serve immediately.

Serves 2.

Penne with Broccoli and Anchovies

The combination of broccoli, roasted garlic, and anchovies gives this dish a rich, savory flavor and plenty of antioxidants. Skip the Parmesan cheese if you want to reduce calories or if you've already had your recommended servings of dairy for the day.

- 1/4 cup olive oil
- 1 pound whole-wheat pasta
- 1/2 pound broccoli or broccoli rabe cut into 1-inch florets
- 3–4 anchovy filets, packed in olive oil
- 2 cloves garlic, sliced
- Pinch red pepper flakes
- 1/4 cup freshly grated, low-fat Parmesan
- Salt substitute and freshly ground pepper, to taste

Heat the olive oil in a deep skillet on medium heat.

In the meantime, prepare the pasta according to package directions for al dente.

Fry the broccoli, anchovies, and garlic in the oil until the broccoli is almost tender and the garlic is slightly browned, about 5 minutes or so.

Rinse and drain the pasta, and add it to the broccoli mixture.

Stir to coat the pasta with the garlic oil.

Transfer to a serving dish, toss with red pepper flakes and Parmesan, and season.

Serves 4.

Quinoa and Broccoli

Originally from the Andes, quinoa is a starch that's quick and easy to cook as well as extremely healthful: it's high in manganese, magnesium, protein, and more. Before cooking quinoa be sure to rinse; otherwise, it may have a bitter flavor.

- 2 tablespoons olive oil
- 1 cup broccoli florets
- 2 cups cooked quinoa
- Zest of 1 lemon
- Salt substitute and freshly ground pepper, to taste

Heat the oil in a large skillet.

Add the broccoli and cook until soft, about 3 minutes.

Remove from heat and add the quinoa and lemon zest. Season and serve.

Serves 4.

Rice Pilaf

Pilaf is a type of rice dish that pairs well with fish and poultry. This dish is seasoned traditionally with cinnamon and raisins, but you can omit these, if you prefer.

- 2 tablespoons olive oil
- 1 medium onion, diced
- 1/4 cup pine nuts
- 1 1/2 cups long-grain brown rice
- 2 1/2 cups chicken stock
- 1 cinnamon stick
- 1/4 cup raisins
- Salt substitute and freshly ground pepper, to taste

Heat the olive oil in a large saucepan over medium heat.

Sauté the onion and pine nuts for 6–8 minutes, or until the pine nuts are golden and the onion is translucent.

Add the rice and sauté for 2 minutes until lightly brown.

Pour the chicken stock into the pan and bring to a boil.

Add the cinnamon and raisins.

Lower the heat, cover the pan, and simmer for 15–20 minutes, or until the rice is tender and the liquid is absorbed.

Remove from the heat and fluff with a fork. Season and serve.

Serves 6.

Seafood Fettuccine

Pasta is delicious and nutritious when topped with fresh vegetables, herbs, and seafood instead of rich sauces and cheese. If you prefer, you can substitute low-sodium, artificial crab for the fresh crab and shrimp.

- 10 ounces dry, whole-wheat fettuccine noodles
- 3 tablespoons garlic, minced
- 1 tablespoon olive oil
- 2 medium tomatoes, cut into bite-sized pieces
- 1 green bell pepper, cut into bite-sized pieces
- 2 tablespoons fresh basil, chopped
- 2 tablespoons fresh oregano, chopped
- 1/2 pound cooked bay shrimp
- 1/2 pound fresh, cooked crab

Boil the fettuccine per package directions.

Meanwhile, combine the garlic and oil in a large, nonstick skillet, and heat gently over medium heat.

Add the tomatoes and pepper to the skillet.

Stir in the basil and oregano, add the shrimp and crab, and cook just until the seafood is heated.

Drain the pasta and stir it into the skillet.

Serves 4.

Spicy Broccoli Pasta Salad

Broccoli can help lower cholesterol, and it's high in vitamins C and K, as well as folate. This salad is perfect for picnics or potlucks.

- 8 ounces whole-wheat pasta
- 2 cups broccoli florets
- 1 cup carrots, shredded
- 1/4 cup plain Greek yogurt
- Juice of 1 lemon
- 1 teaspoon red pepper flakes
- Salt substitute and freshly ground pepper, to taste

Cook the pasta according to the package directions for al dente and drain well.

When the pasta is cool, combine it with the veggies, yogurt, lemon juice, and red pepper flakes in a large bowl, and stir thoroughly to combine.

Taste for seasoning, and add salt substitute and freshly ground pepper as needed.

Can be served at room temperature or chilled.

Serves 2.

Walnut Spaghetti

This delicious, simple dish is traditionally served around Christmastime in Naples, Italy, but it's so easy you'll want to make it all year round! In addition to being tasty, walnuts are high in antioxidants and healthful fats. Toast the walnuts until lightly brown, but don't burn them.

- 1 pound whole-wheat spaghetti
- 1/2 cup olive oil
- 4 cloves garlic, minced
- 3/4 cup walnuts, toasted and finely chopped
- 2 tablespoons low-fat ricotta cheese
- 1/2 cup grated, low-fat Parmesan cheese
- 1/4 cup flat-leaf parsley, chopped
- Salt substitute and freshly ground pepper, to taste

Prepare the spaghetti according to package directions for al dente, reserving 1 cup of the pasta water.

Heat the olive oil in a large skillet on medium-low heat.

Add the garlic and sauté for 1–2 minutes.

Ladle 1/2 cup of the pasta water into the skillet, and continue to simmer for 5–10 minutes.

Add the chopped walnuts and ricotta cheese.

Toss the walnut sauce with the spaghetti in a large serving bowl.

Top with the Parmesan cheese and parsley. Season and serve.

Serves 6.

Wild Mushroom Risotto

Risotto is a type of starchy rice dish that cooks into a creamy consistency. It is classically paired with earthy wild mushrooms and Parmesan cheese. Serve it as a first course, or as a side dish with chicken or pork.

- 2 ounces dried porcini mushrooms (or 6 ounces fresh)
- 5 cups chicken stock
- 2 tablespoons olive oil
- 1 small onion, minced
- 2 cups brown rice
- 1/2 cup grated, low-fat Parmesan cheese
- Salt substitute and freshly ground pepper, to taste

Place the mushrooms in a bowl and cover them with hot water.

Set them aside for 30 minutes.

Drain them, reserving the liquid, and wash them.

Strain the liquid through a sieve lined with cheesecloth.

Add the liquid to the chicken stock.

Heat the chicken stock and mushroom liquid in a small saucepan. When simmering, turn heat to lowest setting.

Heat the oil in a large saucepan over medium heat.

Add the onion and sauté for 3–5 minutes, or until tender.

Stir in the rice and mushrooms and 3/4 cup of the stock.

Continue cooking the rice, stirring almost constantly, and adding more liquid, a ladleful at a time, as soon as the rice absorbs the liquid.

There should always be some liquid visible in the pan.

Cook until the rice is tender, with a slightly firm center, 20–30 minutes.

Remove from the heat, and stir in the Parmesan cheese, a spoonful at a time.

Season to taste and serve.

Serves 6.

POULTRY DISHES

Arroz con Pollo

This dish is easy to prepare and can be adapted to your taste. Add more vegetables, such as artichokes or peas, to boost fiber and decrease calories.

- 4 tablespoons olive oil
- 1 chicken, cut into pieces
- Salt substitute and freshly ground pepper, to taste
- 3 sweet red peppers, coarsely chopped
- 1 onion, chopped
- 2 garlic cloves, minced
- 2 1/2 cups chicken stock
- 1 (14-ounce) can diced tomatoes, drained
- 1 tablespoon paprika
- 1 cup brown rice
- 1/4 cup flat-leaf parsley, chopped

Heat the olive oil in a large skillet on medium-high heat.

Place the chicken in the pan, and cook it 8–10 minutes, or until lightly browned on both sides.

Transfer the chicken to an oven-safe dish, and keep warm in the oven on the lowest setting.

Add salt substitute and freshly ground pepper to taste.

Add the sweet peppers, onion, and garlic to the pan, and cook, stirring frequently, until tender.

Heat the chicken stock in the microwave or a saucepan until simmering.

Add the chicken stock, tomatoes, and paprika to the pan.

Stir in the rice, and place the chicken pieces on top.

Simmer with the lid on for 20–30 minutes, or until the liquid is absorbed and the rice is tender.

Garnish with parsley.

Serve with a green salad or tomato and red onion salad.

Serves 6.

Braised Chicken with Wild Mushrooms

This stew is hearty and satisfying, and can be served with a variety of vegetables or salads. Stews improve with time, so make this the night before you want to serve it.

- 1/4 cup dried porcini or morel mushrooms, or 8 ounces fresh
- 1/4 cup olive oil
- 2–3 slices low-salt turkey bacon, chopped
- 1 chicken, cut into pieces
- Salt substitute and freshly ground pepper, to taste
- 1 small celery stalk, diced
- 1 small, dried red chili, chopped
- 1/4 cup vermouth or white wine
- 1/4 cup tomato puree
- 1/4 cup low-salt chicken stock
- 1/2 teaspoon arrowroot
- 1/4 cup flat-leaf parsley, chopped
- 4 teaspoons fresh thyme, chopped
- 3 teaspoons fresh tarragon

Place the mushrooms in a small bowl and pour boiling water over them.

Allow them to stand for 20 minutes to soften.

Drain and chop, reserving the liquid.

Heat the olive oil in a heavy stew pot on medium heat.

Add the bacon and cook until browned and slightly crisp.

Drain the bacon on a paper towel.

Season the chicken with salt substitute and freshly ground pepper, and add to the oil and bacon drippings.

Cook for 10–15 minutes, turning halfway through the cooking time so that both sides of the chicken are golden brown.

Add the celery and the chopped chili, and cook for 3–5 minutes or until soft.

Deglaze the pan with the wine, using a wooden spoon to scrape up the brown bits stuck to the bottom.

Add the tomato puree, chicken stock, arrowroot, and mushroom liquid.

Cover and simmer on low for 45 minutes.

Add the fresh chopped herbs and cook an additional 10 minutes, until the sauce thickens.

Season with salt substitute and freshly ground pepper to taste.

Serve with wilted greens or crunchy green beans.

Serves 4.

Braised Duck with Fennel Root

Roasted or braised fennel is sweet and mild, and fennel provides a great source of vitamin C, fiber, and potassium. It pairs perfectly with the rich taste of duck, but you can also use chicken, which is leaner and lower in calories.

- 1/4 cup olive oil
- 1 whole duck, cleaned
- 3 teaspoon fresh rosemary
- 2 garlic cloves, minced
- Salt substitute and freshly ground pepper, to taste
- 3 fennel bulbs, cut into chunks
- 1/2 cup sherry

Preheat the oven to 375 degrees.

Heat the olive oil in a large stew pot or Dutch oven.

Season the duck, including the cavity, with the rosemary, garlic, salt substitute, and freshly ground pepper.

Place the duck in the oil, and cook it for 10–15 minutes, turning as necessary to brown all sides.

Add the fennel bulbs and cook an additional 5 minutes.

Pour the sherry over the duck and fennel, cover the pot, and cook in the oven for 30–45 minutes, or until internal temperature of the duck is 140–150 degrees at its thickest part.

Allow duck to sit for 15 minutes before serving.

Serves 6.

Chicken and Potato Tagine

The term "tagine" refers to both the cooking vessel and the finished dish. Use a Dutch oven or casserole dish if you don't have a tagine. Small amounts of meat and poultry are balanced with large servings of vegetables on this diet—but watch your intake of potatoes (remember: one serving per week)!

- 1 chicken, cut up into 8 pieces
- 1 medium onion, thinly sliced
- 3 cloves garlic, minced
- 1/4 cup olive oil
- 1/2 teaspoon ground cumin
- 1/2 teaspoon freshly ground pepper
- 1/4 teaspoon ginger
- Pinch saffron threads
- 1 teaspoon paprika
- Salt substitute, to taste
- 2 cups water
- 3 cups potatoes, peeled and diced
- 1/2 cup fresh, flat-leaf parsley, chopped
- 1/2 cup fresh cilantro, chopped
- 1 cup fresh or frozen green peas

Place the chicken, onion, garlic, oil, and seasonings into a Dutch oven.

Add about 2 cups water and bring to a boil over medium-high heat.

Reduce heat and simmer covered for 30 minutes.

Add the potatoes, parsley, and cilantro, and simmer an additional 20 minutes, or until the potatoes are almost tender.

Add the peas at the last moment, simmering for an additional 5 minutes.

Serve hot.

Serves 6.

Chicken Marsala

The secret to this classic is to pound the chicken breasts thin between two pieces of wax paper, so they cook quickly and evenly. Small servings of meat and large portions of vegetables are easy to achieve with this entree.

- 1/4 cup olive oil
- 4 boneless, skinless chicken breasts, pounded thin
- Salt substitute and freshly ground pepper, to taste
- 1/4 cup whole-wheat flour
- 1/2 pound mushrooms, cleaned and sliced
- 1 cup Marsala
- 1 cup chicken broth
- 1/4 cup flat-leaf parsley, chopped

Heat the olive oil in a large skillet on medium-high heat.

Season the chicken breasts with salt substitute and pepper, and dredge them in flour.

Sauté them in the olive oil until golden brown.

Transfer to an oven-safe plate, and keep warm in the oven on low.

Sauté the mushrooms in the same pan. Add the wine and chicken broth, and bring to a simmer.

Simmer for 10 minutes, or until the sauce is reduced and thickened slightly.

Return the chicken to the pan, and cook it in the sauce for 10 minutes.

Transfer to a serving dish and sprinkle with the parsley.

Serves 4.

Grilled Chicken and Vegetables with Lemon-Walnut Sauce

This grilled chicken and vegetable dish gets a boost from a rich, pureed walnut sauce. Other vegetables, such as artichokes, carrots, eggplant, or endive, can be used in place of or in addition to the zucchini and asparagus.

- 1 cup chopped walnuts, toasted
- 1 small shallot, very finely chopped
- 1/2 cup olive oil, plus more for brushing
- Juice and zest of 1 lemon
- 4 boneless, skinless chicken breasts
- Salt substitute and freshly ground pepper, to taste
- 2 zucchini, sliced diagonally 1/4-inch thick
- 1/2 pound asparagus
- 1 red onion, sliced 1/3-inch thick
- 1 teaspoon Italian seasoning

Preheat a grill to medium-high.

Put the walnuts, shallots, olive oil, lemon juice, and lemon zest in a food processor and process until smooth and creamy.

Season the chicken with salt substitute and freshly ground pepper, and grill on an oiled grate until cooked through, about 7–8 minutes a side or until an instant-read thermometer reaches 180 degrees in the thickest part.

When the chicken is halfway done, put the vegetables on the grill.

Sprinkle Italian seasoning over the chicken and vegetables to taste.

To serve, lay the grilled veggies on a plate, place the chicken breast on the grilled vegetables, and spoon the lemon-walnut sauce over the chicken and vegetables.

Serves 4.

Lebanese Grilled Chicken

This grilled chicken is flavored with baharaat, an Arabic spice mix that includes cumin, paprika, coriander, nutmeg, cloves, cinnamon, and black pepper. The chicken must be marinated in these spices for several hours, or overnight. If you are looking to cut calories, use chicken breasts instead of a whole chicken.

- 1/2 cup olive oil
- 1/4 cup apple cider vinegar
- Juice and zest of 1 lemon
- 4 cloves garlic, minced
- 2 teaspoons salt substitute
- 1 teaspoon Arabic 7 spices
- 1/2 teaspoon cinnamon
- 1 chicken, cut up into 8 pieces

Combine all the ingredients except the chicken in a shallow dish or plastic bag.

Place the chicken in the bag and marinate overnight, or at least for several hours.

Drain, reserving the marinade.

Heat the grill to medium-high.

Cook the chicken pieces for 10–14 minutes, brushing them with the marinade every 5 minutes or so.

The chicken is done when the crust is golden brown and an instant-read thermometer reads 180 degrees in the thickest parts. Remove skin before eating.

Serves 4.

Pomegranate-Glazed Chicken

In this recipe, the pomegranate juice makes a sweet, fruity glaze for boneless, skinless chicken breasts. From start to finish, this dish takes less than 30 minutes to prepare.

- 1 teaspoon cumin
- 1 clove garlic, minced
- Salt substitute and freshly ground pepper, to taste
- 6 tablespoons olive oil, divided
- 6 boneless, skinless chicken breasts
- 1 cup pomegranate juice (no sugar added)
- 2 tablespoons honey
- 1 tablespoon Dijon mustard
- 1/2 teaspoon dried thyme
- 1 fresh pomegranate, seeds removed

Mix the cumin, garlic, salt substitute, and freshly ground pepper with 2 tablespoons of olive oil, and rub into the chicken.

Heat the remaining olive oil in a large skillet over medium heat.

Add the chicken breasts and sauté for 10 minutes, turning halfway through the cooking time, so the chicken breasts are golden brown on each side.

Add the pomegranate juice, honey, Dijon mustard, and thyme.

Lower the heat and simmer for 20 minutes, or until the chicken is cooked through and the sauce reduces by half.

Transfer the chicken and sauce to a serving platter, and top with fresh pomegranate seeds.

Serves 6.

Roast Chicken

Roast chicken may seem intimidating, but it's actually one of the simplest chicken dishes you can make. Remember, small portions of meat and large portions of vegetables are the DASH diet way! Prepare this chicken for a lazy Sunday dinner, and you'll have leftovers for lunch on Monday.

- 1/4 cup white wine
- 2 tablespoons olive oil, divided
- 1 tablespoon Dijon mustard
- 1 garlic clove, minced
- 1 teaspoon dried rosemary
- Juice and zest of 1 lemon
- Salt substitute and freshly ground pepper, to taste

- 1 large roasting chicken, giblets removed
- 3 large carrots, peeled and cut into chunks
- 1 fennel bulb, peeled and cut into 1/2-inch cubes
- 2 celery stalks, cut into chunks

Preheat the oven to 400 degrees.

Combine the white wine, 1 tablespoon of olive oil, mustard, garlic, rosemary, lemon juice and zest, salt substitute, and freshly ground pepper in a small bowl.

Place the chicken in a shallow roasting pan on a roasting rack.

Rub the entire chicken, including the cavity, with the wine and mustard mixture.

Place the chicken in the oven and roast for 15 minutes.

Toss the vegetables with the remaining tablespoon of olive oil, and place around the chicken.

Turn the heat down to 375 degrees, and continue roasting the chicken.

Roast an additional 40–60 minutes, basting the chicken every 15 minutes with the drippings in the bottom of the pan.

Cook chicken until internal temperature reaches 170–180 degrees in between the thigh and the body of the chicken. When you remove the instant-read thermometer, the juices should run clear.

Let the chicken rest for at least 10–15 minutes before serving. On the DASH diet you don't eat the skin.

Serves 4.

Roasted Cornish Hen with Figs

Tiny Cornish hens make an elegant presentation for any special dinner. The figs and white wine add sweetness and depth to this simple dish, and the fresh figs provide a good source of fiber.

- 2 Cornish game hens
- 2 tablespoons olive oil
- 1 tablespoon Herbs de Provence
- Salt substitute and freshly ground pepper, to taste
- 1 pound fresh figs
- 1 cup dry white wine

Preheat the oven to 350 degrees.

Place the Cornish hens in a shallow roasting pan and brush them with olive oil.

Season them liberally with Herbs de Provence, salt substitute, and freshly ground pepper.

Roast the hens for 15 minutes, or until they are golden brown.

Add the figs and white wine and cover the hens with aluminum foil.

Cook an additional 20–30 minutes, or until the hens are cooked through.

Allow to rest for 10 minutes before serving.

Serves 2.

Rosemary Chicken

Quick and easy to make, this chicken dish can be served hot or cold. Try it chilled and sliced with a salad for lunch.

- Canola oil spray
- 1 (12-ounce) skinless chicken breast
- Freshly ground pepper

- 4 medium fresh tomatoes
- 1 tablespoon red wine vinegar
- 2 large sprigs fresh rosemary
- 1/2 cup dry white wine

Preheat the oven to 375 degrees.

Lightly coat an 8-inch glass baking dish with canola oil spray.

Arrange the chicken in the dish, and dust generously with freshly ground pepper.

Cut the tomatoes into quarters, and arrange them around the chicken.

Sprinkle the vinegar over the tomatoes, and then tuck the rosemary in next to the chicken.

Pour the wine over into the dish, cover tightly with foil, and bake for 35 minutes.

Slice the chicken breast into bite-sized pieces, toss with the rest of the ingredients, and serve.

Serves 2.

White Chili

This mild chicken chili is perfect for potlucks and parties. Use any variety of white beans you like, such as great northern or cannellini beans.

- 1 pound boneless, skinless chicken breasts or thighs, cut into 1-inch cubes
- 1 onion, chopped
- 1 tablespoon olive oil
- 2 (15 1/2-ounce) cans white beans, rinsed and drained
- 1 (14 1/2-ounce) can low-salt chicken broth
- 2 (4-ounce) cans green chilies, chopped
- 2 cloves garlic, minced
- 1/2 teaspoon salt substitute
- 1 teaspoon ground cumin
- 1 teaspoon dried oregano
- Salt substitute and freshly ground pepper, to taste
- Fresh cilantro
- Green onions

In a large Dutch oven, sauté the chicken and onion in oil for 5 minutes over medium-high heat.

Add the beans, broth, green chilies, garlic, salt substitute, and spices. Bring to a boil, then lower the heat and simmer for 20 minutes.

Remove from heat and season with salt substitute and freshly ground pepper to taste.

Top each serving with chopped, fresh cilantro, and green onions.

Serves 4.

MEAT DISHES

Afelia

Afelia gets its unique flavor from coriander, cinnamon, and red wine. Serve it with brown rice and a green salad. The following day, leftovers can be stuffed in a whole-wheat pita or wrap.

- 2 pounds boneless pork roast, cut into 2-inch pieces
- 1 cup red wine
- 1 tablespoon crushed coriander seeds
- 1 cinnamon stick
- Salt substitute and freshly ground pepper, to taste
- 1/4 cup olive oil
- 1 cup small white onions, peeled
- 3 bay leaves

Place the pork chunks in a shallow bowl.

Add the red wine, coriander seeds, and cinnamon stick, and marinate for several hours or overnight.

Drain, reserving the liquid, and pat the pork chunks dry with a paper towel.

Season the pork with salt substitute and freshly ground pepper.

Heat the oil in a large stew pot or skillet.

Add the pork and onions, and cook for 8–10 minutes, stirring frequently.

Add the bay leaves, salt substitute, freshly ground pepper, and reserved liquid.

Cover and simmer on low for 2 hours, or until the pork is very tender.

Remove the lid, simmer an additional 15 minutes to thicken the sauce, and serve.

Serves 6.

Beef and Wild Mushroom Stew

Earthy, rich, and full of flavor, this stew is an excellent choice for a simple meal. Serve it with a green salad, vegetable side dish, and whole-wheat bread. For a thriftier option than pricey porcini or morels, substitute oyster or Portobello mushrooms.

- 2 pounds fresh porcini or morel mushrooms
- 1/3 cup olive oil
- 2 pounds lean, boneless beef, cut into 2-inch cubes
- 2 medium onions, finely chopped
- 1 clove garlic, minced
- 1 cup dry white wine
- 1 teaspoon thyme, minced
- Salt substitute and freshly ground pepper, to taste

Wash the mushrooms carefully by soaking them in cold water and swirling them around.

Trim away any soft parts of the mushrooms.

Heat the olive oil in a heavy stew pot over medium-high heat.

Brown the meat evenly on all sides, and set aside on a plate.

Add the onions, garlic, and mushrooms to the olive oil, and cook for 5–8 minutes, or until the onions are tender, stirring frequently.

Add the remaining ingredients and return the browned meat to the pot.

Cover and bring to a boil, then reduce heat to low and simmer.

Simmer for 1 hour, or until the meat is tender and flavorful.

Season with salt substitute and freshly ground pepper to taste.

Serves 8.

Beef Stew

This humble beef stew gets its rich flavor from a red wine marinade, and tastes even better if prepared a day ahead. Serve it with whole-wheat noodles or brown rice.

For the marinade:
- 1 cup red wine
- 1/2 cup olive oil
- 1 medium onion, sliced
- 1 celery stalk, sliced
- 1/4 cup brandy
- 2 cloves garlic, minced
- 3/4 teaspoon dried thyme
- Zest of 1 orange

For the stew:
- 2 pounds lean beef stew or pot roast, cut into 2-inch cubes
- 2 tablespoons olive oil
- Salt substitute and freshly ground pepper, to taste
- 1 tablespoon instant flour
- 6 medium carrots, peeled and cut into 1-inch slices
- 14 small pearl onions, peeled
- 1 (14-ounce) can chopped tomatoes, drained
- 1 cup low-salt olives, pitted

Marinade:

Combine the marinade ingredients in a plastic bag and add beef.

Shake well to coat, and refrigerate for up to 24 hours.

Drain and discard the marinade.

Stew:

In a heavy stew pot, heat the olive oil over medium-high heat.

Season the meat with salt substitute and freshly ground pepper, and toss with flour.

Brown the meat in the oil for 8–10 minutes, stirring frequently until all sides are well browned.

Add the remaining ingredients.

Simmer on low for up to 2 hours, or until the carrots and meat are tender.

Serve stew on a bed of noodles or rice.

Serves 8.

Flank Steak and Blue Cheese Wraps

This snack or lunch dish uses leftover flank steak. Heat the flank steak if you like, or serve it cold. To boost the nutrition of these wraps, add fresh spinach leaves.

- 1 cup leftover flank steak, cut into 1-inch slices
- 1/4 cup red onion, thinly sliced
- 1/4 cup cherry tomatoes, chopped
- 1/4 cup low-salt olives, pitted and chopped
- 1/4 cup roasted red bell peppers, drained and coarsely chopped
- 1/4 cup blue cheese crumbles
- 6 whole-wheat or spinach wraps
- Salt substitute and freshly ground pepper, to taste

Combine the flank steak, onion, tomatoes, olives, bell pepper, and blue cheese in a small bowl.

Spread 1/2 cup of this mixture on each wrap, and roll halfway. Fold the end in, and finish rolling like a burrito.

Cut on a diagonal if you'd like, season to taste, and serve.

Serves 6.

Lamb and Vegetable Bake

This one-dish meal combines lamb with a variety of garden vegetables. Improvise with the vegetables available in your garden or at your local farmer's market, but to maintain the authentic flavor, don't change the seasonings.

- 1/4 cup olive oil
- 1 pound boneless, lean lamb, cut into 1/2-inch pieces
- 2 large red potatoes, scrubbed and diced
- 1 large onion, coarsely chopped
- 2 cloves garlic, minced
- 1 (28-ounce) can diced tomatoes with liquid (no salt added)
- 2 medium zucchini, cut into 1/2-inch slices
- 1 red bell pepper, seeded and cut into 1-inch cubes
- 2 tablespoons flat-leaf parsley, chopped
- 1 teaspoon dried thyme
- 1 tablespoon paprika
- 1/2 teaspoon ground cinnamon
- 1/2 cup red wine
- Salt substitute and freshly ground pepper, to taste

Heat the olive oil in a large stew pot or cast-iron skillet over medium-high heat.

Add the lamb and brown the meat, stirring frequently.

Transfer the lamb to an ovenproof baking dish.

Preheat the oven to 325 degrees.

Cook the potatoes, onion, and garlic in the skillet until tender and transfer them to the baking dish.

Pour the tomatoes, zucchini, and pepper into the pan along with the herbs and spices and simmer for 10 minutes.

Cover the lamb, onions, and potatoes with the tomato and pepper sauce and wine.

Cover with aluminum foil and bake for 1 hour.

Uncover during the last 15 minutes of baking.

Season to taste, and serve with a green salad.

Serves 8.

Lamb Stew

Perfect for a light, spring meal, lamb stew tastes even better the next day.
Serve with a vegetable salad and a whole-wheat baguette.

- 3 carrots, peeled and sliced
- 2 onions, minced
- 2 cups white wine
- 1/2 cup flat-leaf parsley, chopped
- 2 garlic cloves, minced
- 3 bay leaves
- 1 teaspoon dried rosemary leaves
- 1/4 teaspoon nutmeg
- 1/4 teaspoon ground cloves
- 2 pounds boneless lamb, cut into 1-inch pieces
- 1/4 cup olive oil
- 1 package frozen artichoke hearts
- Salt substitute and freshly ground pepper, to taste

Combine the carrots, onion, white wine, parsley, garlic, bay leaves, and seasonings in a plastic bag or shallow dish.

Add the lamb and marinate overnight.

Drain the lamb, reserving the marinade, and pat dry.

Heat the oil in a large stew pot. Brown the lamb meat, turning frequently.

Pour the marinade into the stew pot, cover, and simmer on low for 2 hours.

Add the artichoke hearts and simmer an additional 20 minutes.

Season with salt substitute and freshly ground pepper.

Serves 6.

Pork and Cannellini Bean Stew

This delectable stew is the ultimate budget dish. Hearty and filling, it costs surprisingly little per serving. Serve with brown rice and a salad for a full meal.

- 1 cup dried cannellini beans
- 1/4 cup olive oil
- 1 medium onion, diced
- 2 pounds pork roast, cut into 1-inch chunks
- 3 cups water
- 1 (8-ounce) can tomato paste
- 1/4 cup flat-leaf parsley, chopped
- 1/2 teaspoon dried thyme
- Salt substitute and freshly ground pepper, to taste

Rinse and sort the beans.

Cover them with water, and allow them to soak overnight.

Heat the oil in a large stew pot.

Add the onion, stirring occasionally, until golden brown.

Add the pork chunks and cook 5–8 minutes, stirring frequently, until the pork is browned.

Add the water, and bring to a boil.

Reduce heat and simmer for 45 minutes.

Drain and rinse the beans, and add to the pot.

Add the tomato paste, parsley, and thyme, and simmer an additional 15 minutes, or until the sauce thickens slightly. Season to taste.

Serves 6.

Pork Loin in Dried Fig Sauce

Pork loin is a lean meat and pairs beautifully with fruit or fruity wine. If you can't find dried figs, substitute apricots instead. Both dried figs and apricots are high in fiber.

- 3 teaspoon fresh rosemary
- 1 tablespoon fresh thyme
- Salt substitute and freshly ground pepper, to taste
- 1 (3-pound) pork loin
- 1/2 cup olive oil
- 3 carrots, peeled and sliced
- 1 onion, diced
- 1 garlic clove, minced
- 1 cup dried figs, cut into small pieces
- 1 cup white wine
- Juice of 1 lemon

Preheat the oven to 300 degrees.

Mix the rosemary, thyme, salt substitute, and freshly ground pepper together to make a dry rub. Press the rub into the pork loin.

Heat the olive oil in a skillet.

Add the pork loin, carrots, onion, and garlic, and cook for 15 minutes, or until the pork is browned.

Transfer all to a shallow roasting pan.

Add the figs, white wine, and lemon juice.

Cover with aluminum foil and bake for 40–50 minutes, or until the meat is tender and internal temperature is about 145 degrees.

Transfer the meat to a serving dish, and cover with aluminum foil.

Wait 15 minutes before slicing.

In the meantime, pour the vegetables, figs, and liquids into a blender.

Process until smooth and strain through a sieve or strainer.

Transfer to a gravy dish, or pour directly over the sliced meat.

Serves 6.

Roast Pork Tenderloin

By simply altering the seasonings slightly, this traditional pork tenderloin takes on a decidedly Spanish flair. Remember, the diet allows three to six servings of lean meats per week, depending on your calorie intake. Serve it with red potatoes, or add it to salads, wraps, or sandwiches.

- 2 tablespoons olive oil
- 1 teaspoon Spanish paprika
- 1 teaspoon red wine vinegar
- 1 clove garlic, minced
- 1/2 teaspoon ground cumin
- 1/2 teaspoon ground coriander
- 1/2 teaspoon ginger
- 1/2 teaspoon freshly ground pepper
- 1/4 teaspoon turmeric
- 1 pound pork tenderloin
- Salt substitute and freshly ground pepper, to taste

Combine all the ingredients except the pork tenderloin.

Spread over the meat in a thick paste, cover, and refrigerate for several hours or overnight.

Heat a grill to medium heat, and grill the tenderloin for 10–12 minutes, turning halfway through. An instant-read thermometer should read 145 degrees.

Transfer the meat to a serving platter, and allow it to rest for 15 minutes before slicing.

Season to taste and serve.

Serves 6.

Stuffed Flank Steak

In this dish, flank steak becomes tender through slow cooking, making it the perfect dish for a busy day. Simply prepare it the night before, turn the slow cooker on in the morning, and dinner is ready when you are.

- 2 pounds flank steak
- Salt substitute and freshly ground pepper, to taste
- 1 tablespoon olive oil
- 1/4 cup onion, diced
- 1 clove garlic, minced
- 2 cups baby spinach, chopped
- 1/2 cup dried tomatoes, chopped
- 1/2 cup roasted red peppers, diced
- 1/2 cup almonds, toasted and chopped
- Kitchen twine
- 1/2 cup chicken stock

Lay the flank steak out on a cutting board, and generously season with salt substitute and freshly ground pepper.

Heat the olive oil in a medium saucepan.

Add the onion and garlic.

Cook 5 minutes on medium heat, or until onion is tender and translucent, stirring frequently.

Add the spinach, tomatoes, peppers, and chopped almonds, and cook an additional 3 minutes, or until the spinach wilts slightly.

Let the tomato and spinach mixture cool to room temperature.

Spread the tomato and spinach mixture evenly over the flank steak.

Roll the flank steak up slowly, and tie it securely with kitchen twine on both ends and in the middle.

Brown the flank steak in the same pan for 5 minutes, turning it carefully to brown all sides.

Place it in a slow cooker.

Add the chicken stock to the bottom of the cooker and cover.

Cook on low for 4–6 hours.

Cut into rounds, discarding the twine, and serve.

Serves 6.

Zesty Grilled Flank Steak

Flank steak is a lean cut of meat that benefits from a long, slow marinade. Start marinating the meat the night before, and you're ready to go. Thin slices of lean steak can be served over a salad or pile of fresh vegetables. Make sure you are always eating a larger portion of vegetables than meat at any meal.

- 1/4 cup olive oil
- 3 tablespoons red wine vinegar
- 1 teaspoon dried rosemary
- 1 teaspoon dried marjoram
- 1 teaspoon dried oregano
- 1 teaspoon paprika
- 1 teaspoon freshly ground pepper
- 2 pounds flank steak

Combine the olive oil, vinegar, herbs, and seasonings in a small bowl.

Place the flank steak in a shallow dish, and rub the marinade into the meat.

Cover and refrigerate for up to 24 hours.

Heat a charcoal or gas grill to medium heat (350–375 degrees).

Grill the steak for 18–21 minutes, turning once halfway through the cooking time.

An internal meat thermometer should read 135–140 degrees or medium when the meat is done.

Transfer the meat to a cutting board, and cover with aluminum foil.

Let steak rest for at least 10 minutes.

Slice against the grain very thinly and serve.

Serves 6.

SEAFOOD DISHES

Avocado Halibut

This fish dish has a bit of a kick, so beware of the heat. Serve with sliced, fresh tomatoes and a green salad.

- Canola oil spray
- 2 (6-ounce) halibut fillets
- 2 ripe avocados, peeled and pitted
- 1/2 cup mild, green salsa
- 1/2 cup nonfat, Greek yogurt
- 1 fresh jalapeño, seeded and diced

Preheat the broiler.

Lightly coat a broiler pan with canola oil spray.

Set the fillets on the pan.

Mash the avocados and mix in the salsa, yogurt, and jalapeño.

Warm this mixture in a nonstick saucepan over low heat.

Place the halibut fillets on the broiler pan, and broil for 5 minutes, then turn them over and broil another 4 minutes.

Serve the halibut with the warmed guacamole sauce on top.

Serves 2.

Balsamic-Glazed Black Pepper Salmon

Salmon is a rich and fatty fish that is high in health benefits. When purchasing the fish, choose wild Pacific salmon whenever possible. This particular dish pairs well with a light Pinot Noir.

- 1/2 cup balsamic vinegar
- 1 tablespoon honey
- 4 (8-ounce) salmon filets
- Salt substitute and freshly ground pepper, to taste
- 1 tablespoon olive oil

Heat a cast-iron skillet over medium-high heat.

Mix the vinegar and honey in a small bowl.

Season the salmon filets with the salt substitute and freshly ground pepper; brush with the honey-balsamic glaze.

Add oil to the skillet, and sear the salmon filets, cooking for 3–4 minutes on each side until lightly browned and medium rare in the center.

Let sit for 5 minutes before serving.

Serves 4.

Bouillabaisse

Seafood can be enjoyed a few times a week on the DASH diet. Watch your portions with this classic recipe, which calls for a variety of seafood. Serve over brown rice with a large green salad.

- 1/2 cup olive oil
- 2 onions, diced
- 4 tomatoes, peeled and chopped
- 5 cloves garlic, minced
- 3 pints low-salt fish stock
- 8 small red potatoes, cubed and cooked
- 1 cup white wine
- 1 bunch basil leaves, finely chopped
- 1 tablespoon Tabasco or other hot sauce
- 1 teaspoon dried thyme
- 1/2 teaspoon saffron
- 10 clams, scrubbed
- 10 mussels, scrubbed
- 1 pound shrimp, peeled, deveined, and tails removed
- 1 pound fresh monkfish fillets, cut into chunks
- 1 pound fresh cod, cut into chunks
- 1/2 cup flat-leaf parsley, chopped

Heat the olive oil in a large stockpot over medium-high heat.

Add the onions and cook for 5 minutes, or until the onions are soft and translucent.

Add the tomatoes and garlic, and simmer 5 minutes more.

Add the fish stock, potatoes, wine, basil, hot sauce, thyme, and saffron, and simmer for 20 minutes.

Puree half of this mixture in the blender.

Add the shellfish, shrimp, fish, and parsley, and simmer 20 minutes.

Serve with brown rice.

Serves 8.

Chermoula Salmon

Chermoula is a traditional Moroccan marinade that is typically used with fish. Ingredients include cilantro, a good source of phytonutrients, and parsley, providing high levels of vitamin K. The marinade keeps for up to a week in the refrigerator.

- 1/2 cup olive oil
- 1/2 cup fresh cilantro, chopped
- 1/2 cup fresh flat-leaf parsley, chopped
- 4 garlic cloves, minced
- Juice of 1 lemon
- 1 tablespoon cumin
- 1 tablespoon dried red chili pepper
- 1 tablespoon paprika
- 1 teaspoon salt substitute
- 4 salmon fillets

Preheat the oven to 450 degrees.

Combine all the ingredients except the salmon in a small saucepan.

Heat over medium heat just until the mixture is hot, but do not let it boil. Then let cool to room temperature.

Place the salmon on a baking sheet, and rub the marinade over it.

Cover and refrigerate for up to 4 hours.

Bake for 10–13 minutes, or until the salmon is cooked medium rare and is slightly firm to the touch.

Serves 4.

Clam Spaghetti

*Nothing could be simpler for a weeknight meal than this easy pasta dish.
Clams are rich in iron, protein, omega-3 fatty acids, and vitamin B12. Leave
out the low-salt turkey bacon if you are trying to cut calories.*

- 1/4 cup olive oil
- 4 ounces low-salt turkey bacon
- 1 medium onion, diced
- 1 medium green pepper, seeded and diced
- 4 garlic cloves, minced
- 1/2 cup flat-leaf parsley, chopped
- 1/3 teaspoon cayenne pepper
- Salt substitute and freshly ground pepper, to taste
- 3 dozen or so clams, depending on their size
- 1/2 cup white wine
- 1 pound whole-wheat spaghetti
- 1 lemon, cut into wedges
- 1/2 cup freshly grated, low-fat Parmesan cheese

Heat the olive oil in a large skillet over medium heat.

Add the bacon, onion, pepper, and garlic, and cook until the bacon is cooked through and slightly crisp and the onion is translucent.

Add the parsley, cayenne pepper, salt substitute, and freshly ground pepper, and set aside.

Bring a pot of water to a boil.

Add the clams and boil for 10 minutes, or until they open. Remove the clams from the pot, and shell half of them.

Return the skillet to medium-high heat.

Add the shelled clams to the skillet, along with the remaining clams, white wine, and 2 cups of the liquid used to boil the clams.

Cook the pasta according to package directions for al dente, and place in a large serving dish.

Ladle the clam and bacon mixture over the pasta, and toss to serve.

Garnish with lemon wedges and Parmesan cheese.

Serves 4.

Cod Gratin

A gratin is any dish with a crispy topping of breadcrumbs or cheese. In this tasty dish, cod, leeks, and olives peek out from a light, whole-wheat, breadcrumb crust. Serve with sautéed greens such as spinach, chard, or kale.

- 1/2 cup olive oil, divided
- 1 pound fresh cod
- 1 cup black olives, pitted and chopped
- 4 leeks, trimmed and sliced
- 1 cup whole-wheat breadcrumbs
- 3/4 cup low-salt chicken stock
- Salt substitute and freshly ground pepper, to taste

Preheat the oven to 350 degrees.

Brush 4 gratin dishes with the olive oil.

Place the cod on a baking dish, and bake for 5–7 minutes.

Cool and cut into 1-inch pieces.

Heat the remaining olive oil in a large skillet.

Add the olives and leeks, and cook over medium-low heat until the leeks are tender.

Add the breadcrumbs and chicken stock, stirring to mix.

Gently fold in the pieces of cod. Divide the mixture between the 4 gratin dishes, and drizzle with olive oil.

Season with salt substitute and freshly ground pepper.

Bake for 15 minutes or until warmed through.

Serves 4.

Grilled Bluefish

The citrus in this dish lends it a sunny flavor. If you can find small, whole bluefish, clean and grill them whole. Otherwise, fillets work fine. Bluefish is a good source of niacin, phosphorus, selenium, vitamin B6, and vitamin B12.

- 1 cup olive oil
- 1/2 cup white wine
- 1/4 cup fresh basil leaves, chopped
- Juice and zest of 2 lemons or oranges
- 2–3 garlic cloves, minced
- 1 teaspoon ground cumin
- 1 teaspoon thyme
- 2 pinches cayenne pepper
- 4 bluefish or fish fillets
- Salt substitute and freshly ground pepper, to taste

Combine all the ingredients except the fish in a plastic bag or shallow bowl.

Divide marinade in half, reserving half in the refrigerator and placing the fish in the other half of the marinade.

Refrigerate for at least 1 hour.

Heat the grill to medium-high.

Brush the grates with olive oil.

Grill the fish for 6–8 minutes, turning halfway through the cooking time.

Season with salt substitute and freshly ground pepper to taste.

Warm the reserved marinade and serve with the fish.

Serves 4.

Grilled Herbed Tuna

Tuna is a meaty fish that stands up well to grilling. Just be sure to brush the grill grates with oil before adding the fish so it doesn't stick.

- 2 tablespoons olive oil
- 2 tablespoons fresh basil, chopped
- Juice and zest of 1 lemon
- 2 teaspoons fresh cilantro, chopped
- 1 clove garlic, minced
- Salt substitute and freshly ground pepper, to taste
- 4 tuna steaks, fresh
- 2 tablespoons flat-leaf parsley, chopped

Preheat the grill to medium-high.

Combine all the ingredients except the fish and parsley in a bowl.

Brush each side of the tuna with the herb mixture, and let marinate for at least 30 minutes in the refrigerator.

Grill 8–12 minutes depending on thickness, turning halfway through the cooking time.

Garnish with chopped parsley, season to taste, and serve immediately.

Serves 4.

Halibut with Roasted Vegetables

Halibut is a firm, mild fish that pairs well with a variety of seasonings and vegetables. Here, it's combined with tomatoes and zucchini, but feel free to improvise with what's available in your garden or farmer's market.

- 1/4 cup small white mushrooms, coarsely chopped
- 2 small tomatoes, coarsely chopped
- 1 small white onion, chopped
- 2 zucchini, chopped
- 2 cloves garlic, minced
- 1 teaspoon Herbs de Provence
- 1/2 cup olive oil
- Salt substitute and freshly ground pepper, to taste
- 1 1/2 pounds halibut steak, cut into 6 pieces
- 3 tablespoons fresh tarragon, chopped finely
- Juice of 1 lemon

Preheat the oven to 350 degrees.

Toss the mushrooms, vegetables, and herbs on a large baking sheet with the olive oil, and season with salt substitute and freshly ground pepper.

Roast for 15–20 minutes, or until soft and slightly browned. Do not burn.

Place the halibut steaks on another baking sheet, and season with the tarragon, salt substitute, freshly ground pepper, and lemon juice.

Roast for 10–13 minutes.

Top the halibut steaks with the roasted vegetables.

Serves 6.

Herb-Marinated Flounder

Although dried herbs work in many recipes, fresh herbs are much tastier. Fresh herbs are also a better source of antioxidants than dry herbs. Most herbs grow easily in a pot on your back step, or even a sunny windowsill in your kitchen.

- 1/2 cup lightly packed, flat-leaf parsley
- 1/4 cup olive oil
- 4 garlic cloves, peeled and halved
- 2 tablespoons fresh rosemary
- 2 tablespoons fresh thyme leaves
- 2 tablespoons fresh sage
- 2 tablespoons lemon zest
- Salt substitute and freshly ground pepper, to taste
- 4 flounder fillets

Preheat the oven to 350 degrees.

Place all the ingredients except the fish in a food processor.

Blend to form a thick paste.

Place the fillets on a baking sheet, and brush this paste on them. Refrigerate for at least 1 hour.

Bake for 8–10 minutes, or until the flounder is slightly firm and opaque.

Season with salt substitute and freshly ground pepper.

Serves 4.

Shrimp Salad

Main dish salads are a great way to get many servings of vegetables in one meal. Serve this tasty fare with whole-wheat pita bread for a light lunch or dinner.

For the vinaigrette:

- 1/8 cup red wine vinegar
- Juice of 1 lemon
- 1 small shallot, finely minced
- 1 tablespoon fresh mint, chopped
- 1/4 teaspoon dried oregano
- 1/4 cup olive oil
- Salt substitute and freshly ground pepper, to taste

For the salad:

- 1 pound shrimp, deveined and shelled
- Juice and zest of 1 lemon
- 1 clove garlic, minced
- 2 cups baby spinach leaves
- 1 cup romaine lettuce, chopped
- 1/2 cup grape tomatoes
- 1 medium cucumber, peeled, seeded, and diced
- 1/2 cup low-salt olives
- 1/4 cup low-fat feta cheese

Vinaigrette:

To make the vinaigrette, combine the wine vinegar, lemon juice, shallot, chopped mint, and oregano in a bowl.

Add the oil, whisking constantly for up to 1 minute, or until you create a smooth emulsion, and season with salt substitute and freshly ground pepper.

Refrigerate for 1 hour and whisk before serving if separated.

Salad:

Combine the shrimp with the lemon juice and garlic in a shallow bowl or bag. Marinate for at least 2 hours.

Grill the shrimp in a grill basket or sauté in a frying pan 2–3 minutes until pink.

In a large bowl, toss the greens, tomatoes, cucumber, olives, and feta cheese together.

Toss the shrimp with the salad mixture, and drizzle with the vinaigrette.

Serve immediately.

Serves 4.

VEGETABLE DISHES

Braised Eggplant and Tomatoes

This thick vegetarian ragù is delicious enough to eat over a grain. Getting your daily allowance of vegetables is easy with a dish like this.

- 1 large eggplant, peeled and diced
- Pinch salt substitute
- 1 (15-ounce) can chopped tomatoes and juices
- 1 cup chicken broth
- 2 garlic cloves, smashed
- 1 tablespoon Italian seasoning
- 1 bay leaf
- Salt substitute and freshly ground pepper, to taste

Cut the eggplant into 1/2-inch slices and "salt" both sides to remove bitter juices.

Let the eggplant sit for 20 minutes before rinsing and patting dry.

Cube eggplant.

Put eggplant, tomatoes, chicken broth, garlic, seasoning, and bay leaf in a large saucepot.

Bring to a boil and reduce heat to simmer.

Cover and simmer for about 30–40 minutes until eggplant is tender.

Remove garlic cloves and bay leaf, season to taste, and serve.

Serves 4.

Grilled Eggplant Pesto Stack

Making pesto is a cinch, and it's best to avoid store-bought varieties unless you find a good low-salt version. Eggplant is hearty enough to be a great meat substitute.

For the pesto:
- 1 large bunch basil, or 1 cup tightly packed basil leaves
- 1/2 cup pine nuts, toasted
- 2–3 cloves garlic
- Juice of 1 lime
- 3/4 cup olive oil
- 1/2 cup freshly grated, low-fat Parmesan cheese
- Salt substitute and freshly ground pepper, to taste

For the eggplant:
- 1 medium eggplant, sliced into 1/2-inch thick slices
- 2 tablespoons olive oil

Pesto:

Put the basil, pine nuts, garlic, and lime juice in a food processor, and pulse until you have a thick paste.

Continue to pulse and slowly drizzle in the olive oil until you have a creamy sauce.

Fold in the cheese unless you plan to freeze the pesto.

Season with salt substitute and freshly ground pepper.

Eggplant:

Preheat a grill to medium-high heat.

"Salt" the eggplant on both sides and let rest for 20 minutes to get the bitter juices out.

Rinse the eggplant and pat dry with a paper towel.

Brush the eggplant with 2 tablespoons olive oil, and lay on the grill.

Grill for 5–6 minutes per side, until the eggplant is lightly charred, but still firm.

To serve, layer the grilled eggplant with the pesto on individual plates.

Serves 4.

Grilled Vegetables

Less fat doesn't have to mean less flavor. Here, balsamic vinegar adds pizzazz to a variety of grilled vegetables. Feel free to substitute vegetables.

- 4 carrots, peeled and cut in half
- 2 onions, quartered
- 1 zucchini, cut into 1/2-inch rounds
- 1 red bell pepper, seeded and cut into cubes
- 1/4 cup olive oil
- Salt substitute and freshly ground pepper, to taste
- Balsamic vinegar

Heat the grill to medium-high.

Brush the vegetables lightly with olive oil, and season with salt substitute and freshly ground pepper.

Place the carrots and onions on the grill first because they take the longest.

Cook the vegetables for 3–4 minutes on each side.

Transfer to a serving dish, and drizzle with olive oil and balsamic vinegar.

Serves 4.

Mushroom-Stuffed Zucchini

Fresh zucchini with mushrooms seasoned with garlic, olive oil, parsley, herbs, and spices hardly seems like diet food. These mushroom-stuffed zucchini boats make an easy and impressive dish that is low in calories but still filling. Serve with a piece of fish, or serve alone for lunch.

- 2 tablespoons olive oil
- 2 cups button mushrooms, finely chopped
- 2 cloves garlic, finely chopped
- 2 tablespoons chicken broth
- 1 tablespoon fresh parsley, finely chopped
- 1 tablespoon Italian seasoning
- Salt substitute and freshly ground pepper, to taste
- 2 medium zucchini, cut in half lengthwise

Preheat your oven to 350 degrees.

Heat a large skillet over medium heat, and add the olive oil.

Add the mushrooms and cook until tender, about 4 minutes.

Add the garlic and cook for 2 more minutes.

Add the chicken broth and cook another 3–4 minutes

Add the parsley and Italian seasoning, and season with salt substitute and freshly ground pepper.

Stir and remove from heat.

Scoop out the insides of the halved zucchini and stuff the mushroom mixture into the zucchini.

Put them in a casserole dish, and drizzle a tablespoon of water or broth in the bottom.

Cover with foil and bake for 30–40 minutes until zucchini are tender.

Serve immediately.

Serves 2.

Roasted Balsamic Brussels Sprouts with Pecans

This is a terrific recipe for those who say they don't like Brussels sprouts, as roasting them brings out their sweetness. The vinegar helps by adding a tart flavor as well, and will make getting your daily requirement of vegetables a breeze. Substitute walnuts or almonds for the pecans, if you prefer.

- 20–25 medium-sized Brussels sprouts, quartered
- 2 tablespoons olive oil
- 1 tablespoon balsamic vinegar
- Salt substitute and freshly ground pepper, to taste
- 1/4 cup chopped pecans, toasted

Preheat oven to 400 degrees.

Spread sprouts on a single layer on a baking sheet.

Drizzle with olive oil, vinegar, salt substitute, and freshly ground pepper.

Roast for 15–20 minutes until tender and caramelized.

Top with the toasted pecans and serve.

Serves 4.

Roasted Vegetable Pizza with Alfredo Sauce

This vegetable pizza will satisfy the craving for a food most everyone loves. Experiment with different combinations of roasted vegetables, and you'll never tire of this recipe.

- 1 bunch asparagus, washed and trimmed, cut into 3-inch pieces
- 1 red onion, sliced into half rounds
- 1 red pepper, cored and sliced
- 1 cup mushrooms, sliced
- 1 small eggplant, ends trimmed, cut into quarter rounds
- 2 tablespoons olive oil
- 1/4 cup pizza sauce
- 1 whole-wheat pizza crust
- 1/2 cup grated, low-fat mozzarella cheese
- 1 teaspoon Italian herb blend

Preheat oven to 400 degrees.

Arrange vegetables in 1 or 2 roasting pans, to accommodate a single layer.

Drizzle with olive oil, and toss until evenly coated.

Arrange in single layer, and transfer to the oven.

Roast for 15 to 20 minutes or until tender. Remove from oven.

Spread sauce over the crust in a thin layer.

Arrange vegetables and sprinkle evenly with mozzarella and herbs. (Do not overload the pizza. There will be leftover vegetables and sauce, which can be stored in the refrigerator and used later on sandwiches, salads, or pasta.)

Bake pizza for 5 to 10 minutes, until cheese is melted and crust is crisp.

Serves 4.

Rosemary-Roasted Acorn Squash

When roasted at high heat, the skin of acorn squash becomes soft, tender, and edible. Meanwhile, the benefits of rosemary are many: it is thought to stimulate the immune system, increase circulation, and improve digestion.

- 1 acorn squash
- 2 tablespoons honey
- 2 tablespoons rosemary, finely chopped
- 2 tablespoons olive oil
- Salt substitute, to taste

Preheat oven to 400 degrees.

Cut squash in half, and clean out the seeds.

Slice each half into 4 wedges.

Mix honey, rosemary, and olive oil.

Lay squash on baking sheet, and sprinkle each slice with a bit of the mixture and a touch of salt substitute.

Turn over and sprinkle other side.

Bake for 30 minutes or so until squash is tender and slightly caramelized, turning each slice over halfway through.

Serve immediately.

Serves 4.

Sautéed Crunchy Greens

If you're looking for a super-low-calorie dish, you can't go wrong with greens. There is no other food that is as low calorie and nutrient dense, so enjoy! Plus, the sunflower seeds included in this dish are high in vitamin E, vitamin B1, manganese, copper, tryptophan, magnesium, selenium, and more.

- 3 tablespoons olive oil
- 2 cloves garlic, minced
- 2 large bunches Swiss chard or kale, sliced, stems removed
- Juice from 1/2 a lemon
- Salt substitute and freshly ground pepper, to taste
- 3 tablespoons sunflower seeds

In a large skillet, heat the olive oil, and add the garlic on medium heat.

Sauté for about a minute, and add the Swiss chard.

Cook until wilted, about 2 more minutes.

Add the lemon juice, salt substitute and freshly ground pepper to taste, and sunflower seeds.

Serve and enjoy!

Serves 4.

Stuffed Bell Peppers

Red bell peppers have more nutrients than green or yellow peppers, including plenty of vitamin C and carotenoids, and their nutritional value is best when they are not subjected to high heat. If you've already had your dairy allowance for the day, simply omit the cheese.

- 3/4 cup feta cheese
- 1/2 cup low-salt olives, pitted
- 1/2 cup plain Greek yogurt
- 1/4 cup minced onion
- 1/4 cup olive oil
- 1 teaspoon thyme, finely chopped
- 1/2 teaspoon dried dill weed
- 6 bell peppers, seeded, cored, and cut in half lengthwise

Combine all the ingredients except the bell peppers in a food processor.

Pulse for 30 seconds, or until blended.

Carefully spoon the mixture into the bell peppers.

Refrigerate for up to 4 hours. Drizzle with olive oil before serving.

Serves 6.

Vibrant Green Beans

These green beans make a delicious addition to roasted meats and are a great alternative to bland, green bean dishes. If you prefer, use lemon juice in place of the wine. Whenever possible, use fresh green beans.

- 2 tablespoons olive oil
- 2 leeks, white parts only, sliced
- Salt substitute and freshly ground pepper, to taste
- 1 pound fresh, green string beans, trimmed
- 1 tablespoon Italian seasoning
- 2 tablespoons white wine
- Zest of 1 lemon

Heat the oil over medium heat in a large skillet.

Add leeks and cook, stirring often, until they start to brown and become lightly caramelized.

Season with salt substitute and freshly ground pepper.

Add green beans and Italian seasoning, cooking for a few minutes until beans are tender but still crisp to the bite.

Add the wine and continue cooking until beans are done to your liking and leeks are crispy and browned.

Sprinkle with lemon zest before serving.

Serves 6.

DESSERTS

Banana Cream Pie Parfaits

Nonfat vanilla pudding and graham cracker crumbs make this a simple and healthful treat, with walnuts and bananas providing potassium and omega-3 fatty acids. These parfaits can be prepared ahead of time, making this an easy dessert option for a picnic.

- 1 cup nonfat vanilla pudding
- 2 low-sugar graham crackers, crushed
- 1 banana, sliced
- 1/4 cup walnuts, chopped
- Honey for drizzling

In small parfait dishes or glasses, layer the ingredients, starting with the pudding and ending with chopped walnuts.

You can repeat the layers, depending on the size of the glass and your preferences.

Drizzle with the honey.

Serve chilled.

Serves 2.

Berry Crumble

While this may seem like a decadent dessert, it's actually loaded with antioxidant-filled berries and cholesterol-lowering oats. If you don't have a cast-iron skillet, simply use a casserole dish instead. Use naturally sweet, ripe berries in this easy-to-make dessert.

- 3 cups mixed berries
- 1 cup rolled oats
- 2 tablespoons brown sugar
- 1 tablespoon whole-wheat flour
- 2 tablespoons margarine

Preheat oven to 400 degrees.

In a 10-inch, cast-iron skillet, lay the berries in an even layer.

Mix the oats with the sugar and flour in a large mixing bowl.

Spread the oat mixture evenly on top of the berries.

Crumble with the butter, and bake for 40–50 minutes until top is brown and berries are bubbly.

Serve warm.

Serves 6.

Berry Parfait

Greek yogurt and berries are a combination you can enjoy without guilt!
Either use one type of berry or a medley, and enjoy as a breakfast, snack, or
dessert.

- 1/2 cup fresh berries such as blueberries, raspberries, or blackberries
- 1 cup vanilla-flavored Greek yogurt
- 1/4 cup Crunchy Granola (see breakfast recipes)

Put half the berries in a parfait glass, and top with the yogurt.

Top with the rest of the berries and the granola.

Serve immediately.

Serves 1.

Cocoa and Coconut Banana Slices

Frozen bananas have a creamy consistency that mimics ice cream. Bananas are good for you, too—providing dietary fiber, vitamin C, potassium, and manganese. This dessert makes a great snack for adults and kids alike.

- 1 banana, sliced
- 2 tablespoons unsweetened, shredded coconut
- 1 tablespoon unsweetened cocoa powder
- 1 teaspoon honey

Lay the banana slices on a parchment-lined baking sheet in a single layer.

Put in the freezer for about 10 minutes, until firm but not frozen solid.

Mix the coconut with the cocoa powder in a small bowl.

Roll the banana slices in honey, followed by the coconut mixture.

You can either eat immediately or put back in the freezer for a frozen, sweet treat.

Serves 1.

Cranberry-Orange Cheesecake Pears

For this fruity, creamy treat, use the lightest cream cheese you can find, or substitute low- or nonfat ricotta. On the other hand, pears are very nutritious: a good source of fiber and low in calories. Finally the cranberries and almonds add flavor but can be swapped out for other dried fruit and nuts if you prefer.

- 5 firm pears
- 1 cup unsweetened cranberry juice
- 1 cup freshly squeezed orange juice
- 1 tablespoon pure vanilla extract
- 1/2 teaspoon ground cinnamon
- 1/2 cup low-fat cream cheese, softened
- 1/4 teaspoon ground ginger
- 1/4 teaspoon almond extract
- 1/4 cup dried, unsweetened cranberries
- 1/4 cup sliced almonds, toasted

Peel the pears and slice off the bottoms so that that they sit upright.

Remove the inside cores, and put the pears in a wide saucepan.

Add the cranberry and orange juice, as well as the vanilla extract and cinnamon.

Bring to a boil, and reduce to a simmer.

Cover and simmer on low heat for 25–30 minutes, until pears are soft but not falling apart.

Beat the cream cheese with the ginger and almond extract.

Stir the cranberries and almonds into the cream cheese mixture.

Once the pears have cooled, spoon the cream cheese into them.

Boil the remaining juices down to a syrup, and drizzle over the top of the filled pears.

Serves 5.

Cucumber-Lime Popsicles

Cucumbers have both antioxidant and anti-inflammatory properties, and adults and kids alike love these easy-to-make summer treats.

- 2 cups cold water
- 1 cucumber, peeled
- 1/4 cup honey
- Juice of 1 lime

In a blender, puree the water, cucumber, honey, and lime juice.

Pour into popsicle molds, freeze, and enjoy on a hot summer day!

Serves 4–6.

Frozen Raspberry Delight

You can make a sorbet-style treat with frozen fruit. While truly tasty, this dessert will also help you meet your daily fruit requirement. Swap the peach or mango for a banana, if you prefer.

- 3 cups frozen raspberries
- 1 peach, peeled and pitted
- 1 mango, peeled and pitted
- 1 teaspoon honey

Add all ingredients into a blender and puree, only adding enough water to keep the mixture moving and your blender from overworking itself.

Freeze for 10 minutes to firm up if desired.

Serves 2.

Grilled Fruit

Juicy summer fruit provides hydration in addition to vitamins. These fruits are also delicious drizzled with balsamic vinegar instead of served with cheese and honey.

- 2 peaches, halved and pitted
- 2 plums, halved and pitted
- 3 apricots, halved and pitted
- 1/2 cup low-fat ricotta cheese
- 2 tablespoons honey

Heat your grill to medium heat.

Oil the grates or spray with cooking spray.

Place the fruit cut-side-down on the grill, and grill for 2–3 minutes per side, until lightly charred and soft.

Serve warm with the ricotta and drizzle with honey.

Serves 2.

Pears with Blue Cheese and Walnuts

Fruit, cheese, and nuts are a classic combination regarding flavor but also health—walnuts provide a good source of omega-3 fatty acids, and pears are a good source of fiber. Enjoy this treat as a dessert or healthful snack.

- 1–2 pears, cored and sliced into 12 slices
- 1/4 cup blue cheese crumbles
- 12 walnut halves
- 1 tablespoon honey

Lay the pear slices on a plate, and top with the blue cheese crumbles.

Top each slice with 1 walnut, and drizzle with honey.

Serve and enjoy!

Serves 1.

Red-Wine Poached Pears

Pears are a low-calorie fruit and a good source of fiber. These make a delicious dessert but are also lovely alongside rich dishes as well.

- 2 cups red wine, such as merlot or zinfandel, more if necessary
- 2 firm pears, peeled

- 2–3 cardamom pods, split
- 1 cinnamon stick
- 2 peppercorns
- 1 bay leaf

Put all ingredients in a large pot and bring to a boil.

Make sure the pears are submerged in the wine.

Reduce heat and simmer for 15–20 minutes until the pears are tender when poked with a fork.

Remove the pears from the wine, and allow to cool.

Bring the wine to a boil, and cook until it reduces to a syrup.

Strain and drizzle the pears with the warmed syrup before serving.

Serves 2.

Tropical Sorbet

Fresh fruit is the basis for this very refreshing sorbet. It can also be served as a palate cleanser between courses. Substitute tangerine juice for the orange juice if you seek a more exotic flavor.

- 2 cups fresh pineapple, cut into 2-inch pieces
- 2 cups fresh mango, sliced
- 2 tablespoons honey
- 2 tablespoons freshly squeezed orange juice

Line a jelly roll pan with plastic wrap.

Arrange fruit in 1 layer.

Cover and seal with more plastic wrap and freeze overnight.

Transfer frozen fruit to the food processor, and pulse until finely chopped.

Add honey and orange juice, and process for 30 seconds.

Taste and add more honey if necessary. Blend for 5 minutes or until very smooth, scraping down the sides a few times.

Spoon into a tightly covered container and return to freezer.

Transfer to the refrigerator for 20 minutes before scooping and serving.

Serves 4.

CPSIA information can be obtained at www.ICGtesting.com
Printed in the USA
LVOW12s2108160813

348208LV00001B/266/P